RAPID
ECG
INTERPRETATION
A SELF-TEACHING MANUAL

Prepared By

Ann E. Norman, RN, BA, BSN
Department of Educational and Consulting Services
Los Angeles County-University of Southern California Medical Center

MACMILLAN PUBLISHING C

NEW YORK

Collier Macmillan Publish.

LONDON

Macmillan Publishing Company
866 Third Avenue, New York, New York 10022

Collier Macmillan Canada, Inc.

Collier Macmillan Publishers · London

Library of Congress Cataloging-in-Publication Data

Norman, Ann E.
  Rapid ECG interpretation.
    1. Electrocardiography—PRoblems, exercises, etc.
  2. Arrhythmia—Diagnosis—Problems, exercises, etc.
  I. Title.
  RC683.5.E5N67   1989   616.1'207547   89-12540
  ISBN 0-02-371791-2

Printing: 2 3 4 5 6 7 8 9   Year: 1 2 3 4 5 6 7 8 9 0

*Dedicated with love
to my husband Harry*

ACKNOWLEDGEMENTS

It is my pleasure to express my sincere appreciation to the following people at the Los Angeles County-University of Southern California Medical Center:

Rosemary J. Free, RN, MA, my Director, for encouraging me to seek publication of this book.

Winifred Kataoka, RNC, MA, Instructional Media Consultant, School of Nursing, for creating the art work.

Nellie Cardona, Staff Assistant, for keyboarding the manuscript onto the word processor.

I would also like to express my sincere appreciation to all the people who helped me collect the rhythm strips, especially Eileen Lipp, RN, MSN, Critical Care Instructor and Magdalena Czerkies, Cardiac Technician.

LOS ANGELES COUNTY
UNIVERSITY OF SOUTHERN CALIFORNIA
MEDICAL CENTER
DEPARTMENT OF EDUCATIONAL
AND CONSULTING SERVICES

RAPID ECG INTERPRETATION
A SELF-TEACHING MANUAL

Objectives

Upon completion of this self-teaching manual, the student will be able to:

Interpret those arrhythmias categorized as basic. These basic arrhythmias include the sinus rhythms, atrial ectopics, A-V heart blocks, and junctional and ventricular ectopics.

Recognize appropriate interventions for each of the basic arrhythmias.

RAPID ECG INTERPRETATION
A SELF-TEACHING MANUAL

Instructions to the Learner

To learn Basic Arrhythmias, one must practice doing interpretations. Practice Strips are included in this manual. Answers to the Practice Strips are given in order for you to check your answers as you proceed. Do not just look at the answers—the only way to learn basic arrhythmias is to practice, practice, practice. You will need a pair of ECG calipers to do the measurements. The calipers may be purchased at any technical book store and most stationery stores.

Chapter 9 is a summary of the ECG characteristics, causes, significance and appropriate interventions for each arrhythmia. You will be directed to refer to this chapter as you proceed through the manual.

The final examination consists of twenty rhythm strips. You should be able to interpret these strips and recognize appropriate interventions. Passing score is 75% correct or better.

CONTENTS

I.   FUNCTIONAL ANATOMY

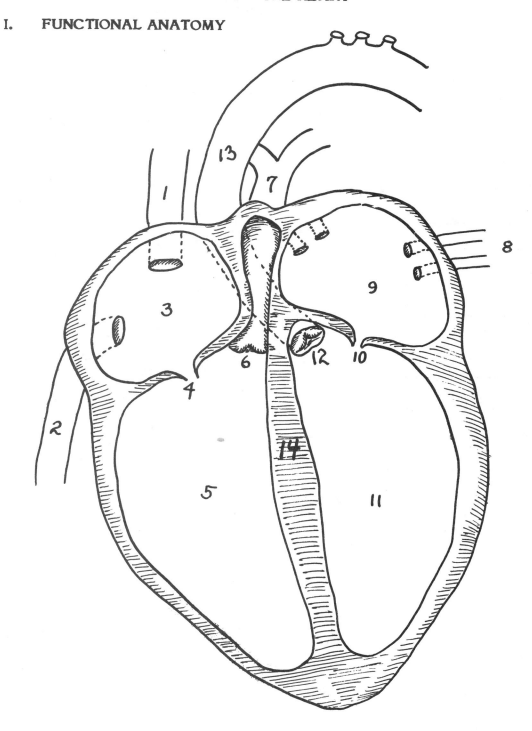

The heart is a double pump. The right side is a low pressure pump that pumps deoxygenated blood to the lungs. The left side is a high pressure pump that pumps oxygenated blood to all other parts of the body.

By way of review, fill in the parts of the heart diagram in the left-hand column; the correct answers are in the right-hand column.

1. _____		1.	Superior vena cava
2. _____		2.	Inferior vena cava
3. _____		3.	Right atrium
4. _____		4.	Tricuspid valve
5. _____		5.	Right ventricle
6. _____		6.	Pulmonic valve
7. _____		7.	Pulmonary artery
8. _____		8.	Pulmonary veins
9. _____		9.	Left atrium
10. _____		10.	Mitral valve
11. _____		11.	Left ventricle
12. _____		12.	Aortic valve
13. _____		13.	Aorta
14. _____		14.	Intraventricular septum

I.   FUNCTIONAL ANATOMY (Cont'd)

You usually think about the heart in terms of the right pump and the left pump. In interpreting Basic Arrhythmias, you need to divide the heart in a different direction.

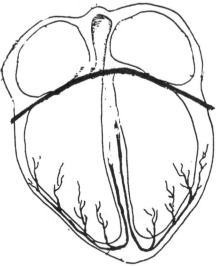

To interpret Basic Arrhythmias we look at the atrial electrical activity and the ventricular electrical activity. The atria are very small compared to the larger ventricles. Therefore, the atrial wave is small on the ECG--the ventricular waves are larger. When atrial and ventricular electrical activity occur simultaneously, we do not see the atrial activity because it is hidden by the larger ventricular waves. On the other hand, when the atria are abnormally enlarged, the atrial waves become larger on the ECG.

II.   ELECTROPHYSIOLOGY

When the cardiac cell is in its resting state, it is said to be POLARIZED. During the polarized state, the inside of the cell is slightly more negative than the outside of the cell represented as follows:

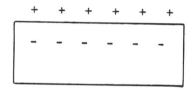

Cardiac cell in
the resting or
POLARIZED STATE

II.   ELECTROPHYSIOLOGY (Cont'd)

The cardiac cell is bathed in an electrolyte solution. An electrical charge builds up in the cell until a point called the threshold is reached. At this point, the cell membrane becomes permeable to sodium (NA^+) and sodium rushes into the cell, carrying its positive charge into the cell:

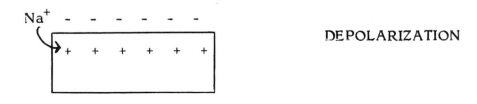

DEPOLARIZATION

Now the inside of the cell is more positive than the outside of the cell--the cell depolarized.

Depolarization (an electrical event) is normally followed by contraction, a mechanical event.

QUESTION

Can we assess the contractile force of the heart using an ECG?

A.   Yes

B.   No

ANSWER

B.   No. On the ECG one can only assess the <u>electrical</u> activity of the heart.

II.   ELECTROPHYSIOLOGY (Cont'd)

Following depolarization, the potassium (K^+) leaves the cell causing the inside to be more negative than the outside. This is called REPOLARIZATION.

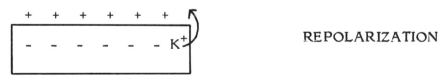

REPOLARIZATION

Repolarization is the recovery process of the cell. The cell must recover and return to the resting state before it can depolarize again.

QUESTION

On the diagram below label the stages of the cardiac cell.

A.   _____

B.   _____

C.   _____

ANSWER

A.   Resting; Polarized
B.   Depolarization
C.   Repolarization

II.   ELECTROPHYSIOLOGY (Cont'd)

It is this movement of the positively charged electrolytes that we see on ECG.

III.   THE CONDUCTION SYSTEM

The conduction system of the heart is composed of specialized fibers that initiate the electrical events and conduct these impulses through the heart.

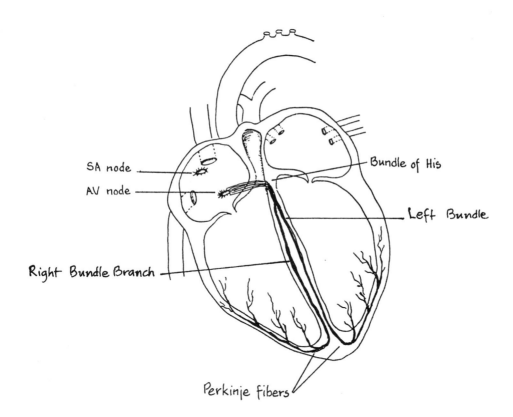

III. THE CONDUCTION SYSTEM (Cont'd)

The picture on the previous page shows:

- The S-A node which initiates the normal rhythmic electrical impulse.

- The A-V node which delays the electrical impulse before it proceeds into the ventricles.

- The junctional bundle which conducts the impulse from the atria to the ventricles.

- The left and right bundle branches which conduct the electrical impulse into the right and left ventricles.

- The Purkinje fibers which conduct the electrical impulse throughout the ventricles.

A. S-A NODE (Sinoatrial node)

The S-A node is the site where the electrical impulse normally begins. The S-A node rhythmically deplorizes and this wave of depolarization spreads through the atria. The S-A node is very small--you do not see its electrical activity on the ECG. You do see the atria depolarize. Depolarization of the atria inscribes the P wave on the ECG.

Following depolarization, the atria repolarize and then return to their resting state before depolarizing again. We do not usually see the atria repolarize on the ECG.

B. A-V NODE (Atrioventricular node)

The A-V node delays the electrical impulse to allow time for the atria to contract while the ventricles are still in diastole. The atria thus can empty their contents into the ventricle before ventricular contraction begins. This synchronization between the atria and the ventricles accounts for approximately 15% of cardiac output. Cardiac output is the amount of blood the heart ejects in one minute.

C. VENTRICULAR CONDUCTION SYSTEM

The electrical impulse then travels into the ventricular system via the A-V junction bundle and down the bundle branches which divide into many small branches called Purkinje fibers.

III. **THE CONDUCTION SYSTEM** (Cont'd)

C. VENTRICULAR CONDUCTION SYSTEM (Cont'd)

The Purkinje fibers are distributed throughout the ventricles. The terminal Purkinje fibers enter the myocardial cell.

The electrical impulse travels very rapidly through the Purkinje fibers resulting in almost immediate transmission of the impulse throughout the entire ventricular system.

The electrical event of depolarization of the ventricle is followed by the mechanical event of muscular contraction. Depolarization of the ventricles inscribes the QRS complex on the ECG.

CHAPTER 2: WAVES, INTERVALS AND MEASUREMENTS

I.   **ECG PAPER**

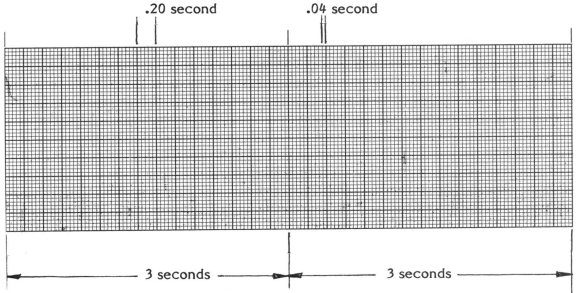

The ECG paper is divided into boxes. There are large boxes that are divided into smaller boxes. There are five small boxes in each large box. Notice the small boxes; each small box is 1 millimeter in both directions. That is, each small box is 1 millimeter high and 1 millimeter wide.

Vertically, each small box is 0.1 millivolt. This is used to standardize the ECG machine. Normal standardization is 10 small boxes or 1 millivolt high. The normal standardization mark is recorded on the ECG paper:

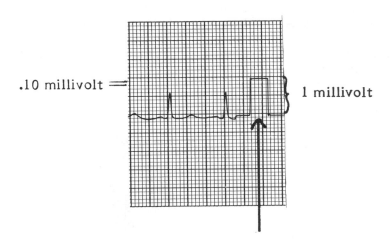

NORMAL STANDARDIZATION MARK

I.   ECG PAPER (Cont'd)

Horizontally each small box represents .04 seconds passage of time.

QUESTION

How much time does <u>one large box</u> represent?

ANSWER

One large box represents .20 seconds. There are five small boxes in one large box (.04 seconds x 5 = .20 seconds).

Five (5) large boxes equals one inch. One inch equals one second.

II.   WAVES

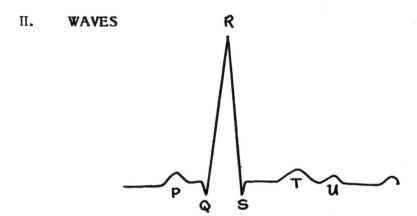

As the stylus moves across the ECG paper, it inscribes a straight line. this is called the isoelectric or the baseline. Electrical activity of the heart causes the stylus to move above and below this isoelectric line. When the stylus inscribes above the line, it is called a positive deflection. When the stylus inscribes below the line, it is called a negative deflection.

Doctor Einthoven arbitrarily named the waves on the ECG as P-Q-R-S-T-U. He could just as easily have named them 1-2-3-4-5-6 or A-B-C-D-E-F. He probably had a sense of humor.

A.   P WAVE

When the atria depolarize, a P Wave is inscribed on the ECG. P waves normally are small (2½ small boxes) and rounded. However, P waves may have other configurations.

P waves may be:

VERY SMALL

II.   **WAVES** (Cont'd)

P waves may be: (Cont'd)

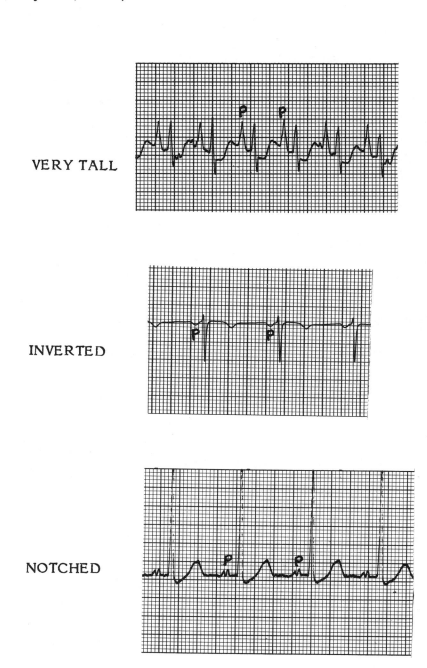

VERY TALL

INVERTED

NOTCHED

II. WAVES (Cont'd)

P waves may be: (Cont'd)

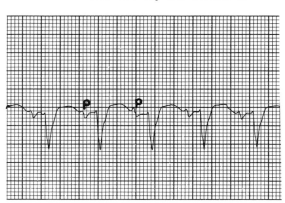

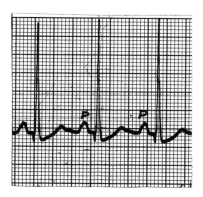

BIPHASIC

(Biphasic means the wave is partly below and partly above the baseline)

Regardless of the shape, size or direction of the P wave, it is always called P WAVE and it represents ATRIAL DEPOLARIZATION.

Atrial depolarization is normally followed by atrial contraction.

QUESTION

Identify the P wave in the following strips.

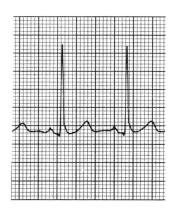

ANSWERS

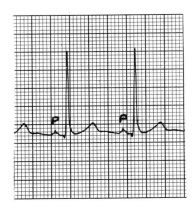

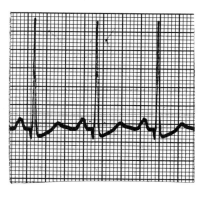

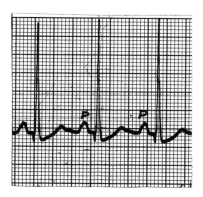

II.   WAVES (Cont'd)

B.   QRS COMPLEX

When the ventricles depolarize, the waves of the complex are inscribed on the ECG. The waves of the complex are the QRS. These waves are specifically named.

Q WAVE: When the first wave of the complex is negative (below the baseline), it is called a Q wave. Q waves MUST BE NEGATIVE and THEY MUST BE THE FIRST WAVE OF THE COMPLEX. Q waves are normally very small.

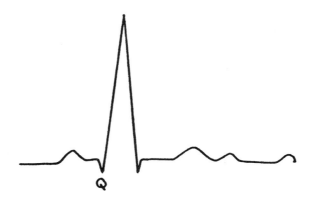

R WAVE: This is the FIRST upward deflection of the complex. R waves are always positive (above the baseline). There is no such thing as "a negative R wave."

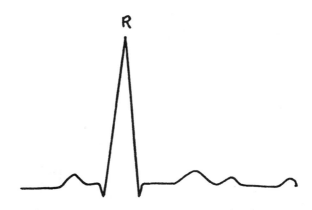

If there are two (2) positive deflections, the second positive one is called R prime (R').

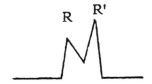

S WAVE: This wave is a negative deflection that follows an R wave.

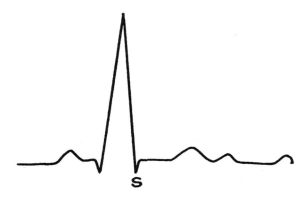

THE DURATION OF THE COMPLEX IS NORMALLY LESS THAN .12 SECONDS

If the wave of the complex is less than 5 millimeters in height or depth (5 little boxes), it is written with a small letter. If the wave is 5 millimeters or more in height or depth, it is written with a capital letter.

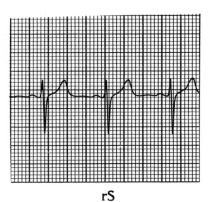

rS

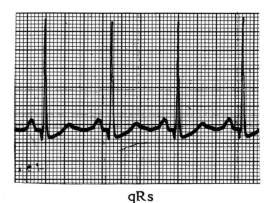

qRs

II.   WAVES (Cont'd)

INSTRUCTIONS

Name the waves of the following complexes and check your answer with the correct answer in the right-hand column:

QUESTION	ANSWER

RS

qR

rS

QUESTION　　　　　　　　　　　　　　　　　　　　　　　　**ANSWER**

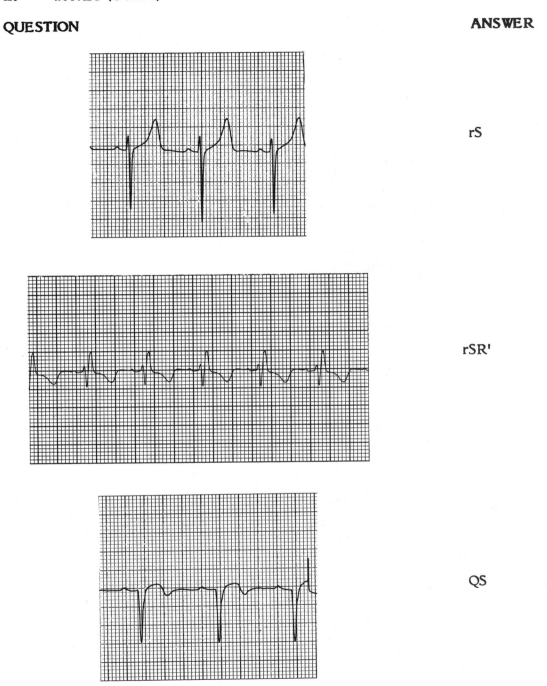

rS

rSR'

QS

When the complex is all negative as in the last strip, it is called QS

II.   WAVES (Cont'd)

The waves of the complex are very specifically named. The complex represents VENTRICULAR DEPOLARIZATION. As you can see from the examples, the complex does not always have a Q wave, an R wave and an S wave. Normally, the complex is less than .12 seconds in duration.

Rhythm disturbances are divided into two categories:

1.   Supraventricular

The pacemaker site is above the ventricle, i.e., in the sinus node, atria or the A-V junction. These rhythms are characterized by normal complexes, unless they are complicated by abnormal conduction through the ventricles. This abnormal conduction through the ventricles is called "aberrant conduction."

2.   Ventricular

Ventricular ectopics produce wide and bizarre QRS complexes.

EXAMPLES

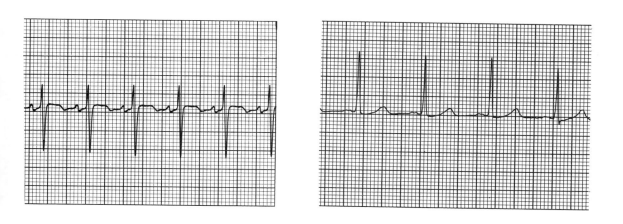

SUPRAVENTRICULAR RHYTHMS WITH NORMAL CONDUCTION
THROUGH THE VENTRICLES

II. WAVES (Cont'd)

EXAMPLES

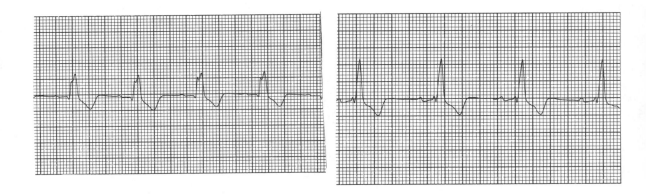

SUPRAVENTRICULAR RHYTHMS WITH ABNORMAL CONDUCTION THROUGH THE VENTRICLES

QUESTION

Supraventricular rhythms will <u>always</u> have normal complexes.

    A.   True
    B.   False

ANSWER

B.   False   Supraventricular rhythms will <u>usually</u> have normal complexes. However, conduction through the ventricles may be delayed causing an abnormal (aberrant) complex on the ECG.

QUESTION

Supraventricular rhythms which conduct abnormally through the ventricles are said to conduct aberrantly.

    A.   True
    B.   False

ANSWER

  A.   True

II.   WAVES (Cont'd)

C.   T WAVES

The T wave represents ventricular repolarization. T waves are usually in the same direction as the complex. T waves normally may be flat or as tall as 10 millimeters. T waves may be biphasic or inverted.

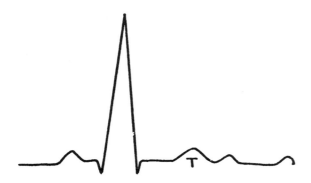

Because they are so labile, T waves do not help interpreting Basic Arrhythmias.

QUESTION:

How many small boxes are ten millimeters?

ANSWER:

Ten. Recall that each small box is one millimeter tall and one millimeter wide.

II.   **WAVES** (Cont'd)

D.   U WAVE

Sometimes there is a wave following the T, before the next P. This wave is the U wave. U waves may be normal or abnormal. Normal U waves probably represent repolarization of the Purkinje fibers.

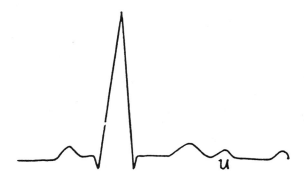

A normal U wave is no more than one-fourth the height of the T wave and is in the same direction as the T wave.

III. PRI INTERVAL (PRI)

The PRI is a very important measurement on the ECG. The PRI is measured from the beginning of the P wave to the beginning of the complex. The PRI represents the time it takes the wave of depolarization to spread through the atria, the A-V node and the A-V junction. The PRI is normally .12 to .20 seconds.

QUESTION

In a normal heart, the PRI on the ECG would be:

    A.   Less than .12 seconds
    B.   .12 to .20 seconds
    C.   More than .20 seconds

ANSWER

B.   The normal PRI is .12 to .20 seconds

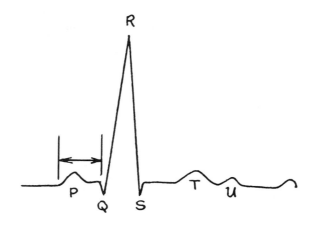

PRI

III. PRI INTERVAL (PRI) (Cont'd)

Also check the PRI's to make sure they are all the same. PRI's are called constant if they are all the same. If the PRI's are not the same, they are called "variable." Note the PR interval on the following strips. These are examples of variable PRI's.

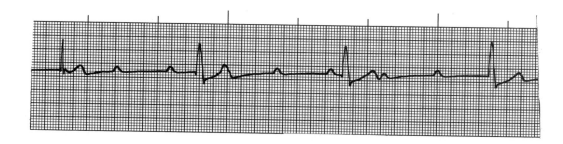

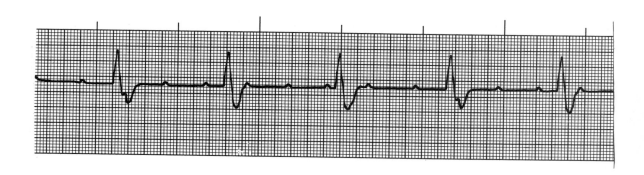

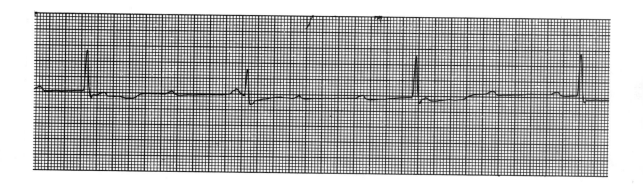

VARIABLE PRI's

IV.   ST SEGMENT

The ST segment is that period on the ECG from the end of the complex to the beginning of the T wave. Normally, this segment is on the isoelectric line.

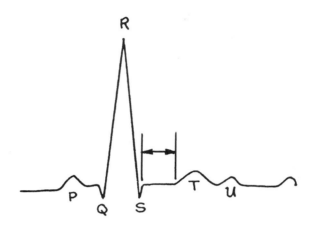

NORMAL ST SEGMENT

If the ST segment is more than 1 millimeter above the isoelectric line, it is called an elevated ST segment. If the ST segment is more than 1 millimeter below the isoelectric line, it is called a depressed ST segment.

IV. ST SEGMENT (Cont'd)

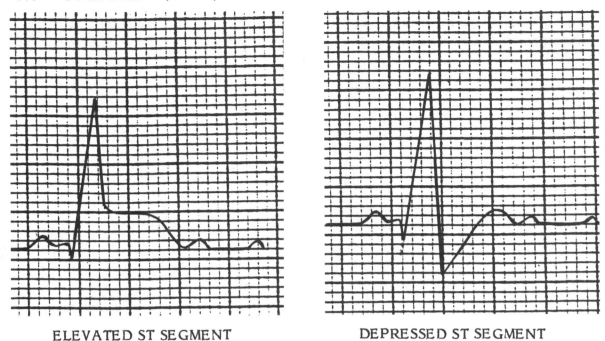

ELEVATED ST SEGMENT   DEPRESSED ST SEGMENT

The ST segment does not help in the interpretation of basic arrhythmias but it is important that you be aware of this area on the ECG!

V. MEASURING INTERVALS

To interpret arrhythmias, you must be able to measure the PRI and the duration of the complex. To make these measurements, you will need ECG calipers. You may purchase ECG calipers for under $10.00.

To measure the PRI, place one point of your calipers at the beginning of the P wave

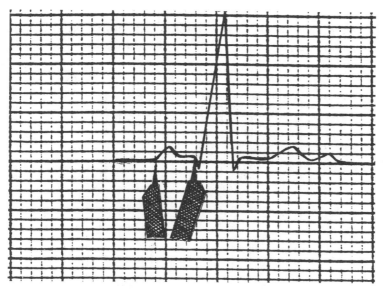

and the other point of the caliper at the beginning of the complex.

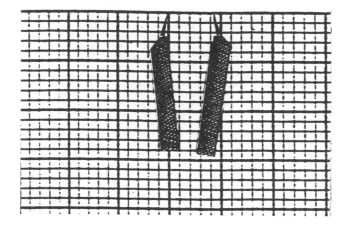

Once you have measured the distance from the beginning of the P wave to the beginning of the complex, pick up your calipers and put them on top of the grid, starting on the large line.

V.   MEASURING INTERVALS (Cont'd)

In the previous example, the distance from the beginning of the P to the beginning of the complex is 4 small boxes. Therefore the PRI is .16 seconds (4 x .04 = .16). Recall that each small box is .04 seconds.

The normal PRI is .12 to .20 seconds. Remember to ascertain if the PRI's are constant or variable.

Measure the complex in the same way. Place one point on the beginning of the complex and the other point on the end of the complex.

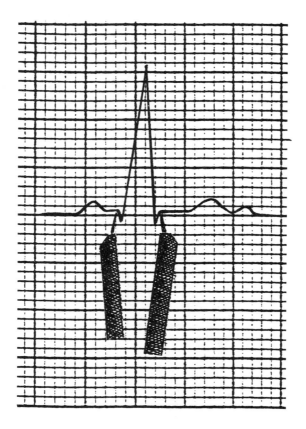

Multiply the number of small boxes by .04 seconds.

In this example, the distance from the beginning of the complex to the end of the complex is 4 small boxes. Therefore, the duration of the complex is .16 seconds (4 x .04 = .16).

INSTRUCTIONS

For each of the following strips in the left-hand column, measure the PRI and the duration of the complex. Also name the waves of the complex. Check your answers with the correct answer in the right-hand column. Don't just look at the answers -- remember, the only way to learn Basic Arrhythmia interpretation is practice, practice, practice. You will not learn if you just look at the answers.

PRACTICE STRIP #1   ANSWER

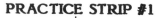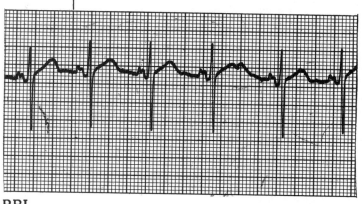

PRI _____
QRS _____

PRI .12. seconds, con-
    stant
RS .08 seconds

PRACTICE STRIP #2   ANSWER

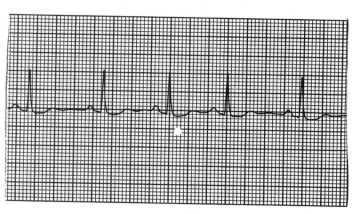

PRI _____
QRS _____

PRI .16 seconds, constant
qRs .06 seconds

PRACTICE STRIP #3

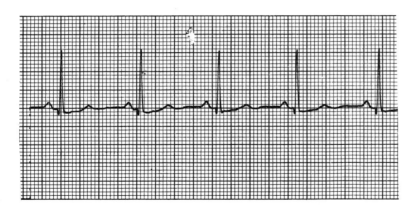

PRI _____

QRS _____

PRI .14 seconds, constant
qR .08 seconds

PRACTICE STRIP #4

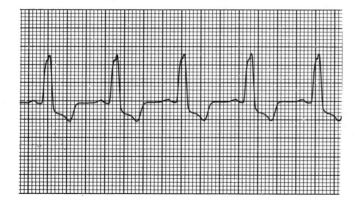

PRI _____

QRS _____

PRI .12 seconds, constant
RS .14 seconds
When the ST segment is elevated or depressed (as it is here) it is not possible to obtain an accurate measurement for the complex-- we just have to "guesstimate" it.

PRACTICE STRIP #5   **ANSWER**

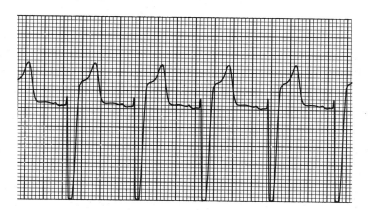

PRI _____
QRS _____

PRI .12 seconds, constant
rS .12 seconds
(Strips #4 & 5 are examples
of supraventricular rhythm
with abnormal (aberrant)
conduction through the ventricles described on page 18.)

PRACTICE STRIP #6   **ANSWER**

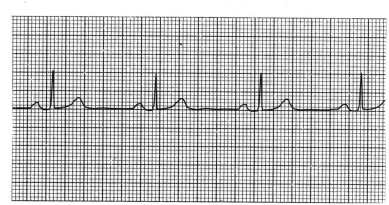

PRI _____
QRS _____
(One-half small box is .02 seconds)

PRI .20 seconds, constant
R .06 seconds

PRACTICE STRIP #7

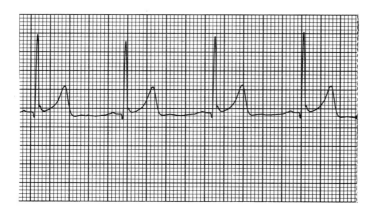

PRI _____
QRS _____

PRI .12 seconds, constant
qR .10 seconds

PRACTICE STRIP #8

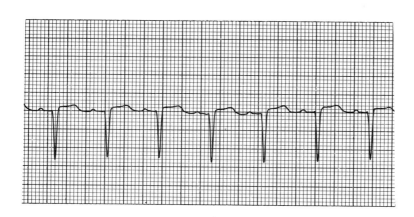

PRI _____
QRS _____

PRI .12 seconds, constant
QS .04 seconds

NOTE:

DO NOT BE CONCERNED IF YOUR PRI OR COMPLEX MEASUREMENTS DIFFER SLIGHTLY FROM THE ANSWER GIVEN. IF YOUR ANSWERS ARE WITHIN ONE SMALL BOX, YOU ARE CORRECT.

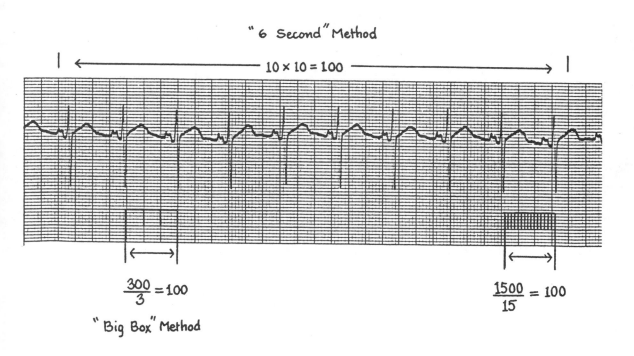

"6 Second" Method

10 × 10 = 100

$$\frac{300}{3} = 100$$

$$\frac{1500}{15} = 100$$

"Big Box" Method

There are many ways to calculate rate on the ECG. We will consider three methods. You probably think of the rate in terms of heart rate. In interpreting ECG's, you not only calculate the heart rate, which is the ventricular rate, you also calculate atrial rate. If you are palpating a pulse or auscultating a chest, you can only assess ventricular rate. Looking at the ECG, you can assess ventricular AND atrial rates. That is one of the advantages of the ECG!!

I.   LARGE BOX METHOD

In one minute, 300 large boxes go through the ECG machine at 25 millimeters per second. Three hundred (300) is the constant in this method. To calculate ventricular rate, measure from complex to complex. To calculate atrial rate, measure from P wave to P wave.

I.   LARGE BOX METHOD (Cont'd)

EXAMPLE

First of all be sure the ventricular rhythm is regular:

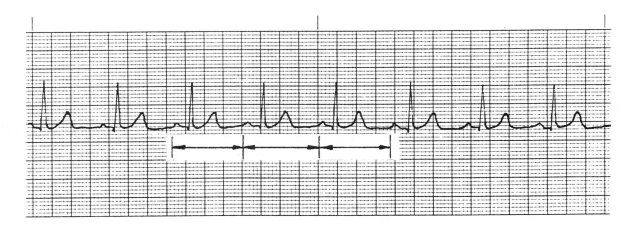

The distance from R to R is the same -- therefore, the ventricular rhythm is regular.

Secondly, be sure the atrial rhythm is regular.

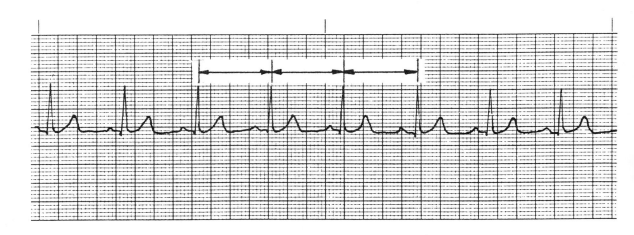

The distance from P wave to P wave is the same -- therefore, the atrial rhythm is regular.

I. LARGE BOX METHOD (Cont'd)

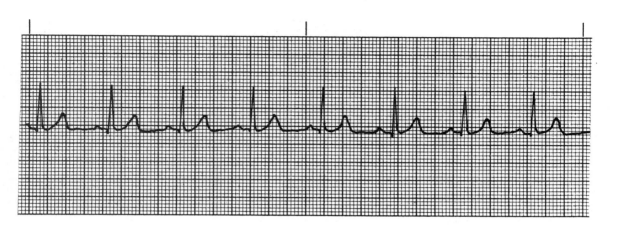

QUESTION

In the above strip, the ventricular rhythm is regular.

A. True
B. False

ANSWER

A. True

QUESTION

In the above strip, the atrial rhythm is regular.

A. True
B. False

ANSWER

A. True

There are 3.8 large boxes between R to R in the above strip. To calculate ventricular rate, divide 3.8 into 300 (300 ÷ 3.8 = 79).

I.   LARGE BOX METHOD (Cont'd)

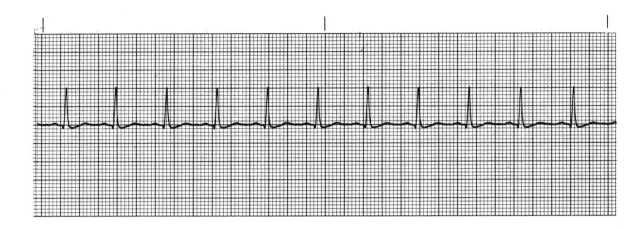

QUESTION

What is the atrial rate in the above strip?

ANSWER

300 ÷ 2.8 = 107. The atrial rate is 107. (There are 2.8 large boxes between P to P.)

QUESTION

What is the ventricular rate in the above strip. There are 2.8 large boxes between R to R.

ANSWER

The ventricular rate is 107 also. HELPFUL HINT: When a P wave is followed by an R wave with a 1:1 conduction and a constant PRI, the atrial and ventricular rates will be the same.

There are 2.8 large boxes between R to R in the above stirp. To calculate ventricular rate, divide 2.8 into 300 (300 ÷ 2.8 = 107).

II.   SMALL BOX METHOD

In one minute, 1500 small boxes go through the ECG machine at 25 mm per second. Fifteen hundred (1500) is the constant in this method. To calculate ventricular rate, measure from complex to complex. To calculate atrial rate, measure from P wave to P wave.

EXAMPLE

First of all, be sure the ventricular rhythm is regular:

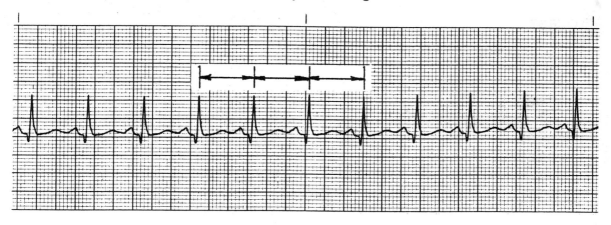

The distance from R to R is the same -- therefore, the ventricular rhythm is regular. Secondly, be sure the atrial rhythm is regular.

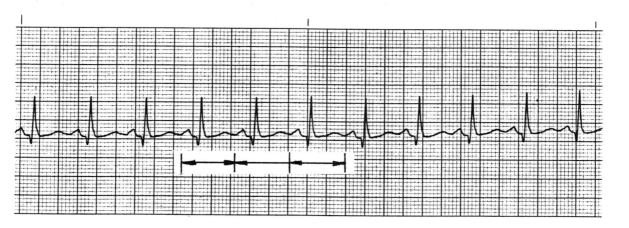

The distance from P to P is regular--therefore the atrial rhythm is regular.

II.   SMALL BOX METHOD (Cont'd)

QUESTION

In the previous strip, what is the ventricular rate?

ANSWER

There are 14 small boxes from R to R. $1500 \div 14 = 107$; the ventricular rate is 107.

QUESTION

In the previous strip, what is the atrial rate?

ANSWER

There are 14 small boxes from P to P. $1500 \div 14 = 107$; the atrial rate is 107.

> Remember the HELPFUL HINT -- whenever a P wave is followed by an R wave with a 1:1 conduction and a constant PRI, the atrial and ventricular rate will be the same.
>
> ANOTHER HELPFUL HINT -- whenever a P wave is followed by an R wave with a 1:1 conduction with a constant PRI, the atrial and ventricular <u>rhythm</u> will be the same.

III: THE SIX-SECOND STRIP METHOD

On the ECG paper, marks appear at three-second intervals. To calculate the ventricular rate, count the number of complexes in six seconds and multiply by 10. (There are 10 six-seconds in one minute.)

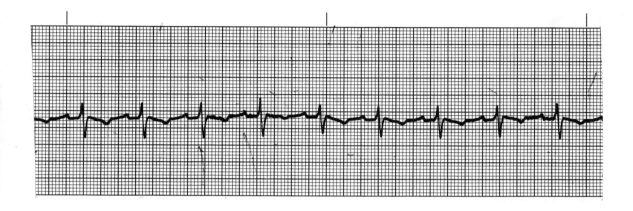

QUESTION

How many complexes are there in the above six-second strip:

ANSWER

Nine (9)

III: THE SIX-SECOND STRIP METHOD

QUESTION

What is the ventricular rate in the previous strip?

ANSWER

90 (9 x 10 = 90)

QUESTION

How many P waves are there in the previous six-second strip?

ANSWER

9

QUESTION

What is the atrial rate?

ANSWER

90 (9 x 10 = 90)

HELPFUL HINT: Whenever the rhythm is irregular, you MUST use this method. The Six-Second Strip Method is the easiest, but you do not always have a six-second strip to work with.

Remember one inch equals one second. Therefore, a six-second strip is six inches.

INSTRUCTIONS

In the following strips, calculate the ventricular and atrial rates using the Big Box or the Small Box Method. Also figure the PRI and the duration of the complex.

PRACTICE STRIP 9   **ANSWER**

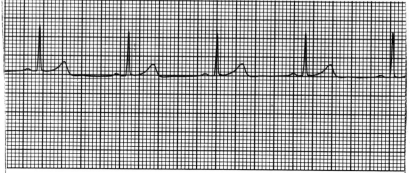

Ventricular Rate _____
Atrial Rate _____
PRI _____   QRS _____

Ventricular Rate = 62
Atrial Rate = 62
PRI = .12 seconds, constant
QRS = .04 seconds

(Did you check the rhythm? Remember to check for regular rhythm before you calculate rates.)

PRACTICE STRIP 10

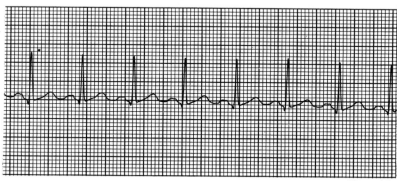

Ventricular Rate _____
Atrial Rate _____
PRI _____   QRS _____

Ventricular Rate = 107
Atrial Rate = 107
PRI = .16 seconds, constant
QRS = .08 seconds

Regular atrial and ventricular rhythms.

NOTE:
DO NOT BE CONCERNED IF YOUR PRI, COMPLEX OR RATE MEASUREMENTS DIFFER SLIGHTLY FROM THE ANSWER GIVEN. IF YOUR ANSWERS ARE WITHIN ONE SMALL BOX, YOU ARE CORRECT.

PRACTICE STRIP #11

ANSWER

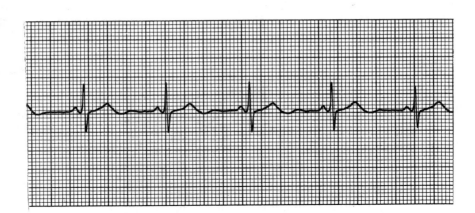

Ventricular Rate _____
Atrial Rate _____
PRI _____   QRS _____

Ventricular Rate = 68
Atrial Rate = 68
PRI = .12 seconds, constant
QRS = .08 seconds

Regular atrial and ventricular rhythm.

PRACTICE STRIP #12

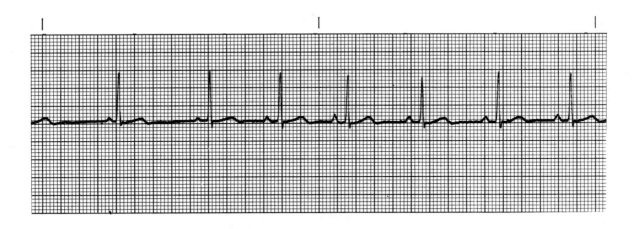

In the above strip, the atrial and ventricular rhythms are irregular, so you must use
the Six-Second Method.

Ventricular Rate _____
Atrial Rate _____
PRI _____   QRS _____

Ventricular Rate = 70
Atrial Rate = 70
PRI = .14 seconds, constant
QRS = .06 seconds

CHAPTER 4: SINUS RHYTHMS

The "pacemaker" of the heart is the place where the depolarization begins. The Sinus Node is the normal pacemaker of the heart. However, there are other potential pacemaker sites:

- Atria

- A-V Junction

- Purkinje Fibers

When the pacemaker site is other than the sinus node, they are called "ectopics." Ectopic pacemakers, like ectopic pregnancies, are abnormal.

QUESTION

The normal pacemaker of the heart is the:

    A.   Sinus Node
    B.   Atria
    C.   A-V Junction
    D.   Ventricle

ANSWER

    A.   Sinus Node

QUESTION

Depolarization which begins in the atria, A-V junction, or ventricles is normal.

    A.   True
    B.   False

ANSWER

    B.   False.   Depolarization which begins anywhere other than the Sinus Node is abnormal. These are called ectopic pacemakers.

Beats that occur early in the cardiac cycle and arise from a pacemaker other than the sinus node are called premature ectopics. Premature ectopics signal irritibility and may need to be treated with a suppressant drug.

Beats that occur late in the cycle and arise from a pacemaker, other than the sinus node, are called escape beats. Escape beats are life-saving mechanisms. Escape beats appear because a higher pacemaker has failed.

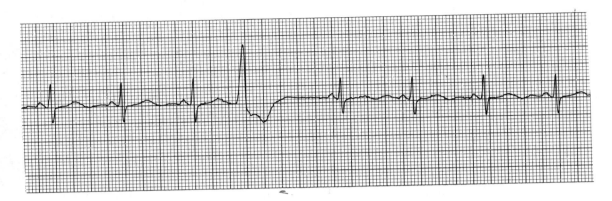

QUESTION

In the above strip, the fourth beat is:
    A.   Premature
    B.   Escape

ANSWER

A. Premature
    The fourth beat is early, it is called "Premature".

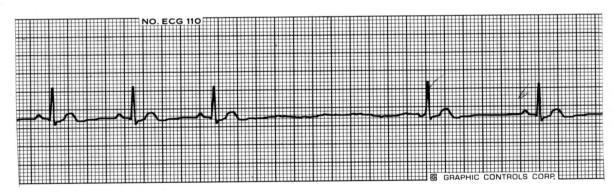

QUESTION

In the above strip, the fourth beat is:
    A.   Premature
    B.   Escape

ANSWER

B. Escape
    The 4th beat is late, it is called "Escape."

The Sinus node is the normal pacemaker of the heart.

REGULAR SINUS RHYTHM

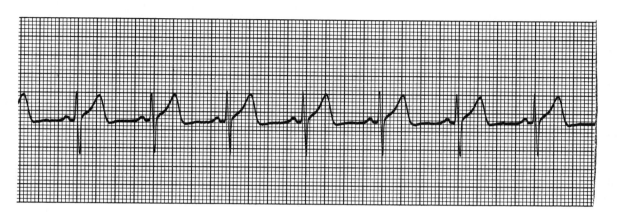

Regular Sinus Rhythm is abbreviated RSR. RSR is synonomous with Normal Sinus Rhythm (NSR). During Regular Sinus Rhythm, the sinus node regularly depolarizes at a rate between 60 to 100 times per minute. This wave of depolarization spreads across the atria creating a P wave on the ECG.

QUESTION

What is the atrial rate on the above strip?

ANSWER

There are 7 P waves in this six-second strip; therefore, the atrial rate is 70.

$$7 \times 10 = 70$$

The A-V node delays the depolarization for the appropriate period of time and then the depolarization spreads through the Bundle of His creating a PRI of .12 to .20 seconds on the ECG.

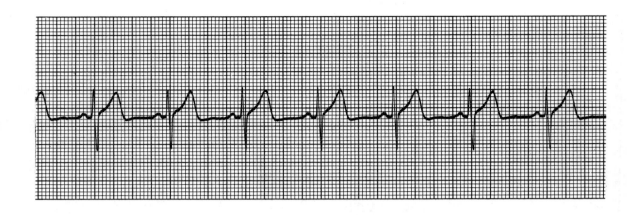

QUESTION

What is the PRI on the above strip?

ANSWER

.12 seconds

QUESTION

Is it constant?

ANSWER

Yes

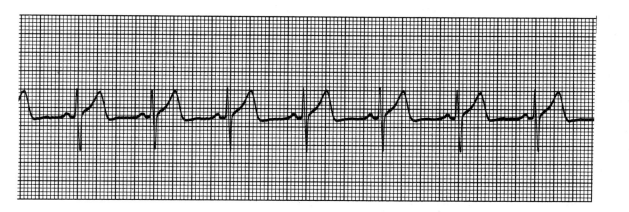

Then the wave of depolarization spreads through the Purkinje fibers causing ventricular depolarization and the formation of the complex on the ECG. The waves of the complex are the QRS. Remember all complexes do not have a Q, an R and an S.

QUESTION

What are the waves of the complex in the above strip?

ANSWER

RS

QUESTION

What is the duration of the complex?

ANSWER

.08 seconds

QUESTION

Conduction through the ventricles is normal on the above strip.

A. True
B. False

ANSWER

A. True. The width of the complex is less than .12 seconds; therefore, conduction through the ventricles is normal.

REGULAR SINUS RHYTHM

ATRIAL RHYTHM:	Regular
VENTRICULAR RHYTHM:	Regular
ATRIAL RATE:	60 to 100 per minute
VENTRICULAR RATE:	60 to 100 per minute
P WAVE:	Present and uniform; one P per complex
PRI:	.12 to .20 seconds; constant
QRS:	Less than .12 seconds

The other sinus rhythms are:

> Sinus Bradycardia
> Sinus Tachycardia
> Sinus Arrhythmia
> Sinus Arrest

The aforementioned sinus rhythms have the same ECG characteristics as Regular Sinus Rhythm EXCEPT one characteristic is different.

For example, Sinus Bradycardia is just like Regular Sinus Rhythm EXCEPT the rate is less than 60.

> Sinus Tachycardia's rate is faster than 100
> Sinus Arrhythmia's atrial and ventricular rhythms are irregular
> Sinus Arrest, the sinus node fails to depolarize when it should.

INSTRUCTIONS

Using the following strip, fill in the blanks in the left-hand column and check your answers with the correct answers in the right-hand column.

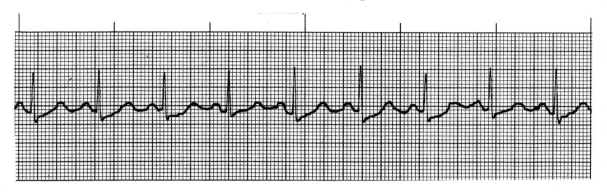

PRACTICE STRIP	ANSWERS
1. Atrial Rhythm: _____	1. Regular
2. Ventricular Rhythm: _____	2. Regular
3. Atrial Rate: _____	3. 90
4. Ventricular Rate: _____	4. 90
5. P Waves: _____	5. Present & uniform; one P per complex
6. PRI: _____	6. .18 seconds, constant
7. QRS: _____	7. .08 seconds
8. Interpretation: _____	8. Regular Sinus Rhythm

The ECG characteristics of Sinus Bradycardia are:

SINUS BRADYCARDIA

ATRIAL RHYTHM:	Regular
VENTRICULAR RHYTHM:	Regular
ATRIAL RATE:	Less than 60 per minute
VENTRICULAR RATE:	Less than 60 per minute
P WAVE:	Present and uniform; one P per complex
PRI:	.12 to .20 seconds; constant
QRS:	Less than .12 seconds

QUESTION

Where is the site of the pacemaker in Sinus Bradycardia?

_____

ANSWER

The sinus node

QUESTION

How fast is the sinus node depolarizing during Sinus Bradycardia?

A. Less than 60 times per minute
B. 60 to 100 times per minute
C. 101 to 160 times per minute
D. More than 160 times per minute

ANSWER

A.   During Sinus Bradycardia, the sinus node is depolarizing less than 60 times per minute. This decrease in heart rate may compromise the patient due to decreased cardiac output.

The only ECG difference between Regular Sinus Rhythm and Sinus Bradycardia is that the atrial and ventricular rates are less than 60 per minute. In Regular Sinus Rhythm, the atrial and ventricular rates are 60 to 100 times per minute.

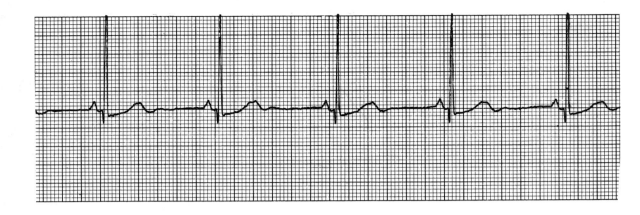

Using the above strip, fill in the following and check your answers with the correct answers in the right-hand column.

PRACTICE STRIP	ANSWERS
1. Atrial Rhythm: _____	1. Regular
2. Ventricular Rhythm: _____	2. Regular
3. Atrial Rate: _____	3. 50
4. Ventricular Rate: _____	4. 50
5. P Waves: _____	5. Present & uniform; one P/complex
6. PRI: _____	6. .14 seconds, constant
7. QRS: _____	7. .08 seconds
8. Interpretation: _____	8. Sinus Bradycardia

The ECG characteristics of Sinus Tachycardia are:

SINUS TACHYCARDIA

ATRIAL RHYTHM:	Regular
VENTRICULAR RHYTHM:	Regular
ATRIAL RATE:	101 to 160
VENTRICULAR RATE:	101 to 160
P WAVE:	Present and uniform; one P per complex
PRI:	.12 to .20 seconds; constant
QRS:	Less than .12 seconds

QUESTION

Where is the site of the pacemaker in Sinus Tachycardia?

─────────────────

ANSWER

The sinus node

QUESTION

How fast is the sinus node depolarizing during Sinus Tachycardia?

A. Less than 60 times per minute
B. 60 to 100 times per minute
C. 101 to 160 times per minute
D. More than 160 times per minute

ANSWER

C. During Sinus Tachycardia, the sinus node is deplarizing 101 to 160 times per minute. The only ECG difference between Regular Sinus Rhythm and Sinus Tachycardia is that during Sinus Tachycardia the atrial and the ventricular rates are between 101 and 160 times per minute.

QUESTION

What are the atrial and ventricular rates during Regular Sinus Rhythm?

ANSWER

60 to 100 times per minute

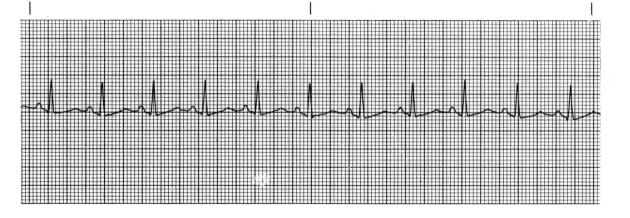

Using the above strip, fill in the following and check your answers with the correct answers in the right-hand column.

PRACTICE STRIP	ANSWERS
1. Atrial Rhythm: _____	1. Regular
2. Ventricular Rhythm: _____	2. Regular
3. Atrial Rate: _____	3. 110
4. Ventricular Rate: _____	4. 110
5. P Waves: _____	5. Present & uniform; one P/complex
6. PRI: _____	6. .14 seconds, constant
7. QRS: _____	7. .08 seconds
8. Interpretation: _____	8. Sinus Tachycardia

The ECG characteristics of Sinus Arrhythmia are:

SINUS ARRHYTHMIA

ATRIAL RHYTHM:	Irregular
VENTRICULAR RHYTHM:	Irregular
ATRIAL RATE:	60 to 100
VENTRICULAR RATE:	60 to 100
P WAVE:	Present and uniform; one P per complex
PRI:	.12 to .20 seconds; constant
QRS:	Less than .12 seconds

QUESTION

Where is the site of the pacemaker in Sinus Arrhythmia? _____

ANSWER

The sinus node

QUESTION

In Sinus Arrhythmia, the rhythm of the atria and ventricles is <u>irregular</u>?

A. True
B. False

ANSWER

A.   True.   The only ECG difference between Regular Sinus Rhythm and Sinus Arrhythmia is the Rhythm. Sinus Arrhythmia is Irregular; Regular Sinus Rhythm is Regular.

QUESTION

How fast is the Sinus Node depolarizing during Sinus Arrhythmia?

A.   Less than 60 times per minute
B.   60 to 100 times per minute
C.   101 to 160 times per minute
D.   More than 160 times per minute

ANSWER

B.   In Sinus Arrhythmia, the Sinus Node is depolarizing 60 to 100 times per minute.

NOTE:

If the sinus node is depolarizing less than 60 times per minute, the interpretation would be Sinus Bradycardia with Arrhythmia. If the rhythm is Sinus Arrhythmia and the sinus node is depolarizing 101 to 160 times per minute, the interpretation would be Sinus Tachycardia with Arrhythmia.

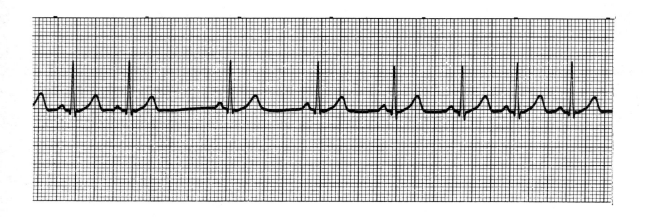

Using the above strip, fill in the following and check your answers with the correct answers in the right-hand column.

PRACTICE STRIP	ANSWERS
1. Atrial Rhythm: _____	1. Irregular
2. Ventricular Rhythm: _____	2. Irregular
3. Atrial Rate: _____	3. 80
4. Ventricular Rate: _____	4. 80
5. P Waves: _____	5. Present & uniform; one P/complex
6. PRI: _____	6. .12 seconds, constant
7. QRS: _____	7. .08 seconds
8. Interpretation: _____	8. Sinus Arrhythmia

The ECG characteristics of Sinus Arrest are:

SINUS ARREST

ATRIAL RHYTHM: Irregular due to the arrest

VENTRICULAR RHYTHM: Irregular due to the arrest

ATRIAL RATE: Slowed due to the arrest

VENTRICULAR RATE: Slowed due to the arrest

P WAVE: Absent during the sinus arrest

PRI: Unable to measure during the arrest

QRS: Absent during the arrest; an ectopic pacemaker may escape to depolarize the ventricle

QUESTION

What happens to the sinus node during Sinus Arrest?

_____

ANSWER

Due to excessive vagal tone and other reasons, the sinus node fails to depolarize and is said to have arrested.

Sinus Arrest is synonomous with Sinus Pause.

The outstanding ECG characteristic of Sinus Arrest is the absence of a P wave (and its complex) when it is expected. During Sinus Arrest an ectopic pacemaker may escape to depolarize the ventricle.

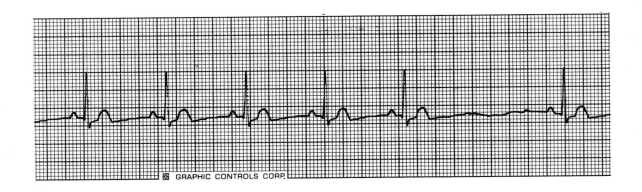

GRAPHIC CONTROLS CORP.

Using the above strip, fill in the following and check your answers with the correct answers in the right-hand column.

PRACTICE STRIP

1. Atrial Rhythm: _____

2. Ventricular Rhythm: _____

3. Atrial Rate: _____

4. Ventricular Rate: _____

5. P Waves: _____

6. PRI: _____

7. QRS: _____

8. Interpretation: _____

ANSWERS

1. Regular except for the pause

2. Regular except for the pause

3. 60

4. 60

5. Present & uniform; one P/complex; absent during the pause

6. .16 seconds, constant

7. .08 seconds

8. RSR with Sinus Arrest

You have now learned the characteristics of the rhythms that originate in the sinus node. On the following practice strips calculate the atrial and ventricular rhythms, the atrial and ventricular rate, the status of the P wave, the duration of the PRI and the ventricular complex. Then interpret the strip. You are reminded to make the measurements; do not just look at the answers. Refer to Chapter 9, page 254 to 261 for the causes, significance and appropriate intervention for the sinus rhythms. The answers to the following practice strips begin on page 62.

PRACTICE STRIP #1

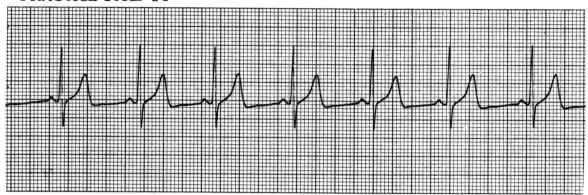

PRACTICE STRIP #2

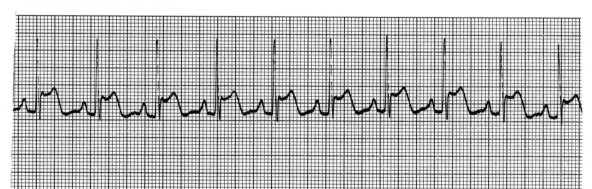

PRACTICE STRIP #3

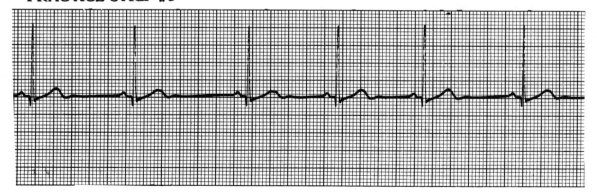

PRACTICE STRIP #4

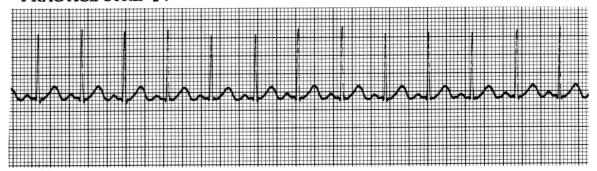

PRACTICE STRIP #5

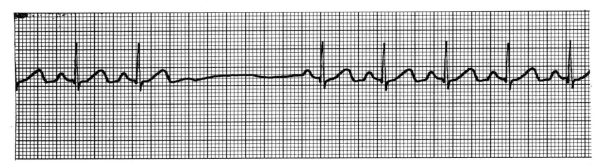

PRACTICE STRIP #6

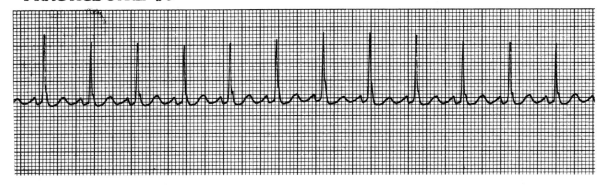

PRACTICE STRIP #7

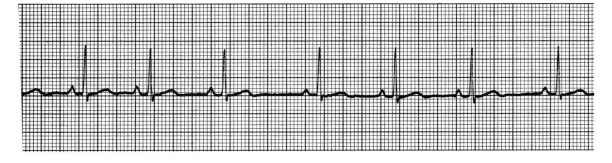

PRACTICE STRIP #8

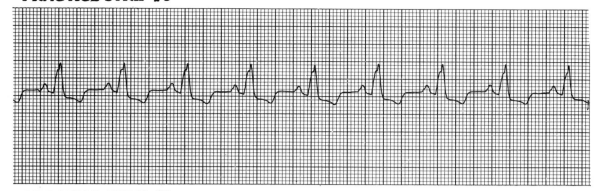

PRACTICE STRIP #9

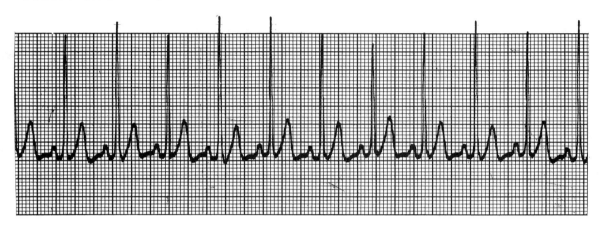

ANSWERS TO PRACTICE STRIPS

PRACTICE STRIP #1

Atrial Rhythm:	Regular
Ventricular Rhythm:	Regular
Atrial Rate:	70
Ventricular Rate:	70
P Waves:	P waves present, one P/complex, uniform
PRI:	.12 seconds and constant
QRS:	.08 seconds
Interpretation:	Regular Sinus Rhythm (RSR)

PRACTICE STRIP #2

Atrial Rhythm:	Regular
Ventricular Rhythm:	Regular
Atrial Rate:	100
Ventricular Rate:	100
P Waves:	P waves present, one P/complex, uniform
PRI:	.18 seconds and constant
QRS:	.08 seconds
Interpretation:	Regular Sinus Rhythm (RSR--notice the elevated ST segment)

PRACTICE STRIP #3

Atrial Rhythm:	Irregular
Ventricular Rhythm:	Irregular
Atrial Rate:	60
Ventricular Rate:	60
P Waves:	P waves present, one P/complex
PRI:	.12 seconds and constant
QRS:	.08 seconds
Interpretation:	Sinus Arrhythmia

ANSWERS TO PRACTICE STRIPS

PRACTICE STRIP #4

Atrial Rhythm:	Regular
Ventricular Rhythm:	Regular
Atrial Rate:	130
Ventricular Rate:	130
P Waves:	P waves present, one P/complex, uniform
PRI:	.14 seconds and constant
QRS:	.06 seconds
Interpretation:	Sinus Tachycardia

PRACTICE STRIP #5

Atrial Rhythm:	Regular except for the pause after the second beat
Ventricular Rhythm:	Regular except for the pause after the second beat
Atrial Rate:	70
Ventricular Rate:	70
P Waves:	P waves present, one P/complex, uniform
PRI:	.20 seconds and constant
QRS:	.08 seconds
Interpretation:	Regular Sinus Rhythm with Sinus Arrest

PRACTICE STRIP #6

Atrial Rhythm:	Regular
Ventricular Rhythm:	Regular
Atrial Rate:	120
Ventricular Rate:	120
P Waves:	P waves present, one P/complex, uniform
PRI:	.12 seconds and constant
QRS:	.08 seconds
Interpretation:	Sinus Tachycardia

ANSWERS TO PRACTICE STRIPS

PRACTICE STRIP #7

Atrial Rhythm:	Irregular
Ventricular Rhythm:	Irregular
Atrial Rate:	70
Ventricular Rate:	70
P Waves:	P waves present, one P/complex, uniform
PRI:	.16 seconds and constant
QRS:	.06 seconds
Interpretation:	Sinus Arrhythmia

PRACTICE STRIP #8

Atrial Rhythm:	Regular
Ventricular Rhythm:	Regular
Atrial Rate:	90
Ventricular Rate:	90
P Waves:	P waves present, one P/complex, uniform
PRI:	.16 seconds and constant
QRS:	.12 seconds
Interpretation:	Regular Sinus Rhythm with Aberrant Ventricular Conduction

PRACTICE STRIP #9

Atrial Rhythm:	Regular
Ventricular Rhythm:	Regular
Atrial Rate:	110
Ventricular Rate:	110
P Waves:	P waves present, one P/complex, uniform
PRI:	.12 seconds and constant
QRS:	.08 seconds
Interpretation:	Sinus Tachycardia

CHAPTER 5: ATRIAL ARRHYTHMIAS

Four atrial arrhythmias are generally described:

- Premature Atrial Contractions

- Atrial Tachycardia

- Atrial Flutter

- Atrial Fibrillation

These atrial arrhythmias arise from an irritable focus in the atria. The atrial arrhythmias are categorized depending on how fast the irritable focus is firing.

PREMATURE ATRIAL CONTRACTION (PAC)

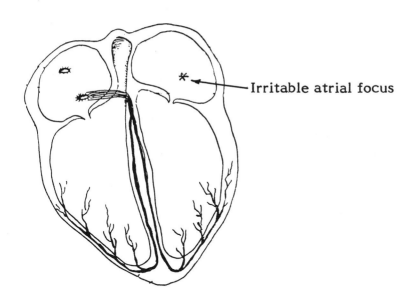

Irritable atrial focus

When this irritable focus fires it will depolarize the atria in a different manner than the sinus node; therefore, the P wave of the PAC will look different than the P wave of the sinus beats. The P wave of the PAC is called P prime (P').

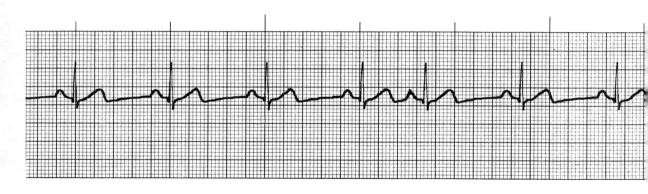

QUESTION

In the above strip, which beat is early?

A. 2nd
B. 5th

ANSWER

B. The 5th beat is early.

Note the P waves <u>(P')</u> of the fifth beat. Can you see it looks different than the other P waves <u>on</u> the strip? The other P waves originate from the sinus node. The fifth P wave originates from an irritable focus in the atria.

The two hallmarks of PAC's are:

1. These beats are early (premature).

2. The P wave (P') looks different than the sinus P wave.

QUESTION

What is the interpretation of the above strip?

ANSWER

Regular Sinus Rhythm with one PAC.

EXAMPLE

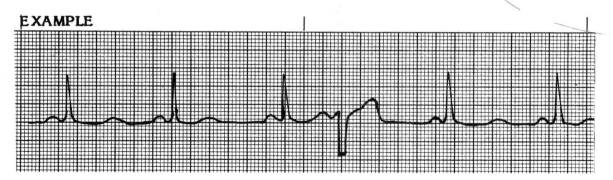

On the above strip, the 4th beat is early and it has a P' -- the two hallmarks of a PAC!

QUESTION

What is the interpretation of the above strip?

ANSWER

Regular Sinus Rhythm with one PAC

The PAC conducted aberrantly (abnormally) to the ventricle. Notice the complex of the P' looks different from the sinus complexes. P'AC's that conduct aberrantly may be mistaken for a Premature Ventricular Contraction (PVC). One way to differentiate between a P'AC with aberrancy and a PVC is the presence or absence of a compensatory pause.

To measure a compensatory pause, measure the distance between three sinus beats (1-2-3 on the strip below).

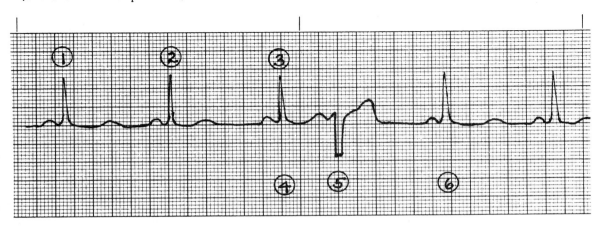

Then compare that distance between three beats, one of which includes the premature beat (4-5-6).

Can you see the distance is NOT the same? When the distance is NOT the same, it is called a NONCOMPENSATORY PAUSE. PAC's usually have a noncompensatory pause.

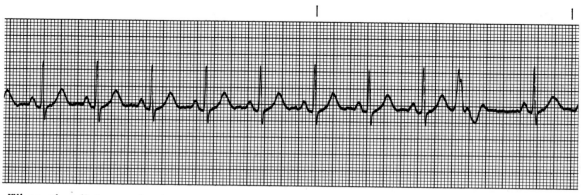

When the distance is the same, it is called a COMPENSATORY PAUSE.

QUESTION

In the above strip, which complex is premature?

ANSWER

The ninth complex

QUESTION

The pause following the premature complex is:

    A.   Compensatory
    B.   Noncompensatory

ANSWER

A. There is a compensatory pause. This premature beat is a <u>PVC</u>. PVC's usually have a compensatory pause.

In Review:

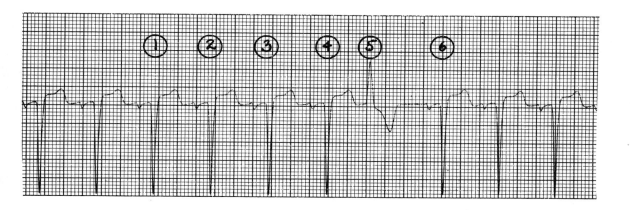

Measure the distance between three sinus beats (1-2-3).

Compare that distance with three other beats, one of which includes the premature (4-5-6). In this case, the distance is the same. When the distance is the same, it is called a compensatory pause.

QUESTION

What is the interpretation of the above strip.

ANSWER

Regular Sinus Rhythm with one PVC

CHAPTER 5: ATRIAL ARRHYTHMIAS (Cont'd)

The ECG characteristics of Premature Atrial Contractions (PAC) are:

PREMATURE ATRIAL CONTRACTIONS

ATRIAL RHYTHM: PAC's will cause the underlying sinus rhythm to be irregular when they occur

VENTRICULAR RHYTHM: Irregular due to the PAC's

ATRIAL RATE: May be increased due to PAC's

VENTRICULAR RATE: May be increased if the PAC is conducted. Decreased if the PAC is not conducted.

P WAVE: P wave of the PAC is early and looks different than the sinus P wave. These early P's are called P prime (P').

PRI: The P'RI is the same as or longer than the PRI of the sinus beat.

QRS:
- May be normal and look like the sinus complexes.
- May be abnormal (aberrant) and look different than the sinus complexes
- May be absent. P' do not always conduct to the ventricle.

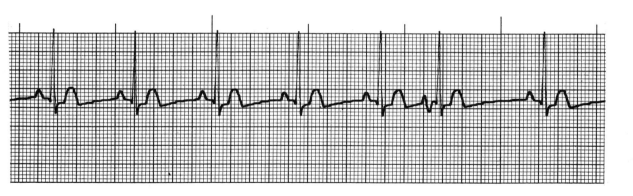

Using the above strip, fill in the following and check your answers with the correct answers in the right-hand column.

PRACTICE STRIP	ANSWERS
1. Atrial Rhythm: _____	1. Regular except for the 6th beat
2. Ventricular Rhythm: _____	2. Regular except for the 6th beat
3. Atrial Rate: _____	3. 70
4. Ventricular Rate: _____	4. 70
5. P Waves: _____	5. Present; one P/complex. The P wave of 6th beat looks different than the other P waves
6. PRI: _____	6. .16 seconds, constant
7. QRS: _____	7. .10 seconds
8. Interpretation:. _____	8. Regular Sinus Rhythm with one PAC

QUESTION

How was the PAC on the previous strip conducted?

A. Normal
B. Abnormal
C. Nonconducted

ANSWER

B. Normal

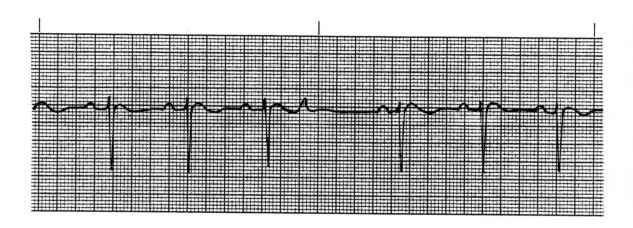

On the above strip, notice the pause after the third beat. Can you see the P' that did not conduct? This is an example of a nonconducted PAC.

QUESTION

What is the interpretation of the above strip.

ANSWER

Regular Sinus Rhythm (the sinus is firing at a rate of 75) with a nonconducted PAC.

In Review:

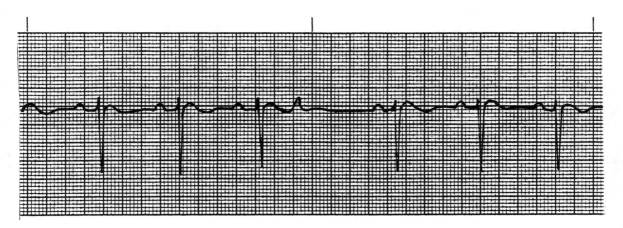

The Sinus Rate is 75. However, due to the pause, the overall rate for 6 seconds is only 60. You can see if the patient is having frequent nonconducted PAC's, the heart rate would be decreased.

QUESTION

Name the two hallmarks of PAC's

ANSWER

A.   PAC's are early

B.   P wave of the PAC (P') looks different than the sinus P waves.

QUESTION

Name three ways PAC's may be conducted to the ventricles.

ANSWER

A.   Normal
B.   Abnormal (aberrant)
C.   Nonconducted

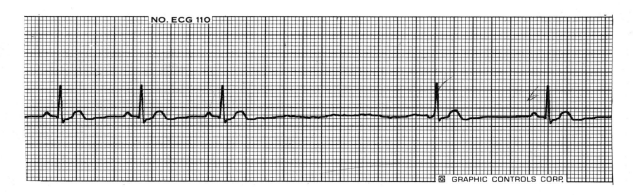

In the above strip, the sinus node arrested after the third complex. Notice the complex that ends the arrest (the fourth complex on the strip).

QUESTION

Did the fourth complex originate from the sinus node?

A.   Yes
B.   No

ANSWER

B.   No

QUESTION

How do you know that the fourth complex did not originate from the sinus node?

ANSWER

Because it does not have a P wave before the complex.

The fourth complex in the above strip is an example of a Junctional Escape Beat. The sinus node arrested for enough time to allow a lower pacemaker to escape. Escape beats are life-saving mechanisms of the heart. Recall the difference between a premature beat such as a PAC and an escape beat. A premature beat occurs due to irritability. Escape beats are life-saving mechanisms that occur because a higher pacemaker has failed.

ATRIAL TACHYCARDIA

Five or more PAC's in a row constitute a run of Atrial Tachycardia. Atrial Tachycardia usually has a sudden beginning and a sudden end. Another word for sudden is "paroxysmal." Atrial Tachycardia is called Paroxysmal Atrial Tachycardia and is abbreviated PAT. The atrial rate in Atrial Tachycardia is 150 to 250. When the atrial rate is rapid, it does not always conduct to the ventricle. This is called a physiological block. Physiological blocks are good! Think about it. If you have an atrial rate of 200, would you want every one to conduct to the ventricle? Of course not--a ventricular rate of 200 is not healthy for humans!

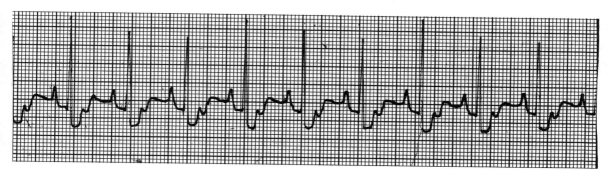

QUESTION

On the above six-second strip, what is the atrial rate?

A. 100
B. 150
C. 200

ANSWER

C. 200! Did you only get 100? If so, you were not counting all the P waves. Let me show you the P waves:

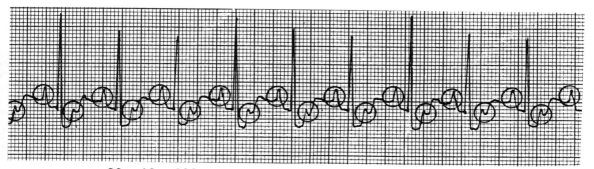

20 x 10 = 200

The atrial rate is 200. The ventricular rate is half that because not every P conducted to the ventricle. Physiological block is present. The interpretation of this strip is Atrial Tachycardia 2:1 (or PAT 2:1). 2:1 means that there are two P's for every one complex.

The ECG characteristics of Atrial Tachycardia are:

ATRIAL TACHYCARDIA

ATRIAL RHYTHM: Regular

VENTRICULAR RHYTHM: Regular

ATRIAL RATE: 150 to 250

VENTRICULAR RATE: Equal to or less than the atrial rate. If the conduction is 1:1 the atrial and ventricular rates would be the same. If there is a physiological block, the ventricular rate would be less than the atrial rate.

P WAVE: Present, but they may be difficult to see.

PRI: .12 to .20 seconds, constant

QRS: Less than .12 seconds

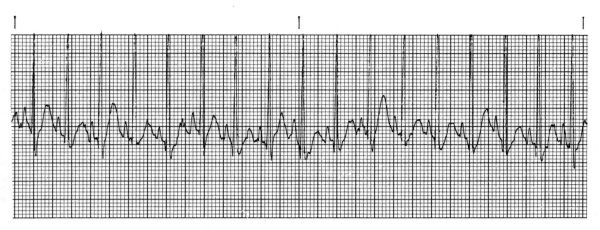

Using the above strip, fill in the left-hand column and check your answers with the correct answers in the right-hand column.

QUESTION	ANSWER
1. Atrial Rhythm: _____	1. Regular
2. Ventricular Rhythm: _____	2. Regular
3. Atrial Rate: _____	3. 170
4. Ventricular Rate: _____	4. 170
5. P Waves: _____	5. Present; one P/complex.
6. PRI: _____	6. .12 seconds, constant
7. QRS: _____	7. .08 seconds
8. Interpretation: _____	8. Atrial Tachycardia (PAT)

ATRIAL FLUTTER

In Atrial Flutter, the irritable focus in the atria is firing even faster than in Atrial Tachycardia.

QUESTION

How fast are the atria depolarizing in Atrial Tachycardia?

A.   60 to 100 times per minute
B.   101 to 160 times per minute
C.   150 to 250 times per minute
D.   Over 300 times per minute

ANSWER

C.   The atria depolarize 150 to 250 times per minute in Atrial Tachycardia.

In Atrial Flutter, the atria depolarize 250 to 350 times per minute. At that fast of an atrial rate, conduction is usually not one to one (1:1).

In untreated Atrial Flutter, the conduction is usually 2:1. The conduction ratio may be 3:1, 4:1, 5:1, 6:1, 7:1, or 8:1. The conduction ratio may vary, in which case it is called "Variable Atrial Flutter."

EXAMPLE: ATRIAL FLUTTER 4:1

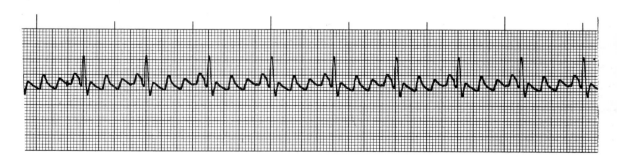

CHAPTER 5:   ATRIAL ARRHYTHMIAS (Cont'd)

ATRIAL FLUTTER

You may have thought the previous strip was 3:1.   You must remember to count the flutter wave that gets lost in the complex.

In Atrial Flutter, the atria continually flutter -- they do not stop.

On the ECG, the atrial pattern may be interrupted by the complex, but you still count it.

There are no P waves.   The atrial activity is called flutter and these are called Flutter waves (F waves).

QUESTION

Do you measure a PRI in Atrial Flutter?

    A.   Yes
    B.   No

ANSWER

B.   No.   You cannot measure a PRI unless you have a P wave.   There is no P wave in Atrial Flutter; therefore, there is no PRI.

The ECG CHARACTERISTICS OF ATRIAL FLUTTER:

ATRIAL FLUTTER

ATRIAL RHYTHM: Regular

VENTRICULAR RHYTHM: Regular or Irregular if the conduction is variable (changes)

ATRIAL RATE: 250 to 350 times per minute (usually 300)

VENTRICULAR RATE: Depends on the conduction ratio

P WAVE: Absent: Flutter waves are present

PRI: Unable to measure

QRS: Less than .12 seconds

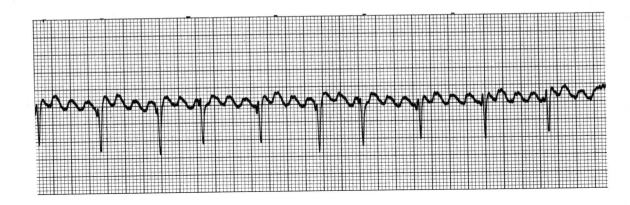

Using the above strip, fill in the left-hand column and check your answers with the correct answers in the right-hand column.

QUESTION	ANSWER
1. Atrial Rhythm: _____	1. Regular
2. Ventricular Rhythm: _____	2. Irregular
3. Atrial Rate: _____	3. 300
4. Ventricular Rate: _____	4. 90
5. P Waves: _____	5. Absent; Flutter waves are present
6. PRI: _____	6. Unable to measure
7. QRS: _____	7. .06 seconds
8. Interpretation: _____	8. Atrial Flutter with variable conduction

CHAPTER 5: ATRIAL ARRHYTHMIAS (Cont'd)

In Atrial Flutter you should always state the ratio because that tells you the approximate heart rate. The <u>atrial rate</u> range in Atrial Flutter is 250 to 350 -- it is usually close to 300. So if you say Atrial Flutter 1:1, you know you are dealing with a serious ventricular tachycardia. Atrial Flutter 2:1 tells you that the patient has a heart rate around 150. Atrial Flutter 4:1 tells you not to worry -- the patient's heart rate is around 75 beats per minute. (300 ÷ 4 = 75.)

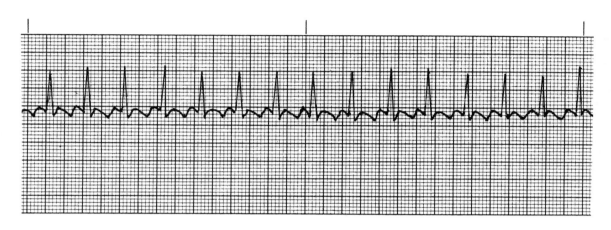

Using the above strip, fill in the left-hand column and check your answers with the correct answers in the right-hand column.

PRACTICE STRIP	ANSWERS
1. Atrial Rhythm: _____	1. Regular
2. Ventricular Rhythm: _____	2. Regular
3. Atrial Rate: _____	3. 300
4. Ventricular Rate: _____	4. 150
5. P Waves: _____	5. Absent, Flutter waves present
6. PRI: _____	6. Unable to measure
7. QRS: _____	7. .08 seconds
8. Interpretation: _____	8. Atrial Flutter 2:1

In Atrial Flutter 2:1, the Flutter waves are difficult to see because every other one is interrupted by a complex. A good rule to remember is any time you have a ventricular rate around 150, think of Atrial Flutter and then look for the Flutter waves. Of course, a ventricular rate of 150 is NOT always Atrial Flutter, but you have a better chance of SEEING the Flutter waves if you LOOK for them.

ANOTHER HINT: Sometimes it is easier to see the Flutter waves if you turn the strip upside down. Try that on the preceding examples of Atrial Flutter.

ATRIAL FIBRILLATION

Now, the irritable focus in the atria has become very rapid -- faster than 350. The atrial activity is so fast we cannot count it and it no longer elicits a regular ventricular response. The uneven, irregular atrial activity is called atrial fibrillation. These fibrillatory waves on the ECG are called f waves.

The atrial activity during atrial fibrillation may appear on the ECG as follows:

A.

B.

C.

A. is called coarse fibrillation

B. is called fine fibrillation

C. is called isoelectric fibrillation

In any case, there are no definite P waves in Atrial Fibrillation.

The hallmarks of Atrial Fibrillation are:

- No definite P wave

- Irregular ventricular rhythm

The ECG characteristics of Atrial Fibrillation are:

ATRIAL FIBRILLATION

ATRIAL RHYTHM: No identifiable P wave

VENTRICULAR RHYTHM: Irregular

ATRIAL RATE: Faster than 350, but you cannot measure it

VENTRICULAR RATE: May be slow, normal or rapid

P WAVE: Absent

PRI: Unable to measure

QRS: Less than .12 seconds

When the Ventricular rate is less than 100, it is called controlled Atrial Fibrillation. When the Ventricular rate is more than 100, it is called uncontrolled Atrial Fibrillation. Clinically, the difference between controlled and uncontrolled is that the physician may need to treat uncontrolled Atrial Fibrillation to slow the ventricular rate. With Controlled Atrial Fibrillation, the patient probably will not be hemodynamically compromised and no treatment will be necessary. Remember, we treat the patient, not the ECG!

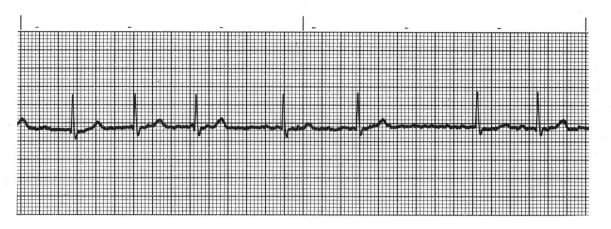

Using the above strip, fill in the left-hand column and check your answers with the correct answers in the right-hand column.

PRACTICE STRIP	ANSWERS
1. Atrial Rhythm: _____	1. Unable to measure
2. Ventricular Rhythm: _____	2. Irregular
3. Atrial Rate: _____	3. Unable to measure
4. Ventricular Rate: _____	4. 70
5. P Waves: _____	5. Absent, fibrillatory wave present
6. PRI: _____	6. Unable to measure
7. QRS: _____	7. .10 seconds
8. Interpretation: _____	8. Atrial Fibrillation, Controlled

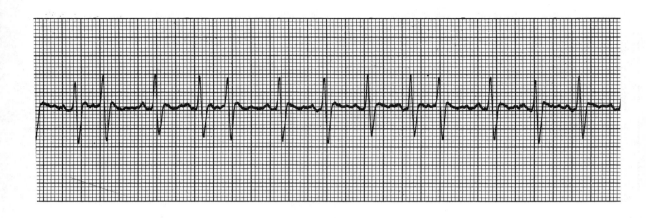

Using the above strip, fill in the left-hand column and check your answers with the correct answers in the right-hand column.

PRACTICE STRIP	ANSWERS
1. Atrial Rhythm: _____	1. Unable to measure
2. Ventricular Rhythm: _____	2. Irregular
3. Atrial Rate: _____	3. Unable to measure
4. Ventricular Rate: _____	4. 130
5. P Waves: _____	5. Absent, fibrillatory waves present
6. PRI: _____	6. Unable to measure
7. QRS: _____	7. .10 seconds
8. Interpretation: _____	8. Atrial Fibrillation, Uncontrolled

CHAPTER 5: ATRIAL ARRHYTHMIAS (Cont'd)

In review the four atrial arrhythmias are:

- Premature Atrial Contractions (PAC's)

- Atrial Tachycardia (PAT)

- Atrial Flutter

- Atrial Fibrillation

These atrial arrhythmias are ectopics caused by irritability.

You have now learned the characteristics of the rhythms that originate in the sinus node and the atrial ectopic arrhythmias. On the following practice strips calculate the atrial and ventricular rhythms, the atrial and ventricular rates, the status of the P wave, the duration of the PRI and the ventricular complex. Then interpret the strip. You are reminded to make the measurements; do not just look at the answers. Refer to Chapter 9 page 262 to 265 for the causes, significance and appropriate interventions for the atrial arrhythmias.

The following practice strips consist of rhythms and arrhythmias orginating from the sinus node and the atria. Answers begin on page 93.

PRACTICE STRIP #10

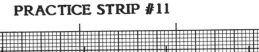

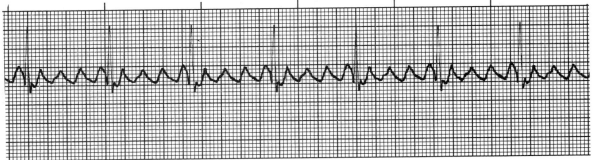

PRACTICE STRIP #11

PRACTICE STRIP #12

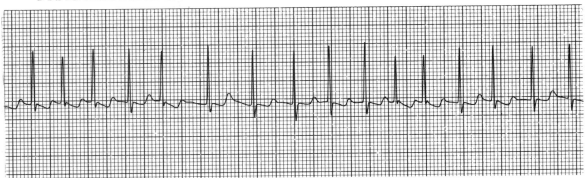

PRACTICE STRIP #13

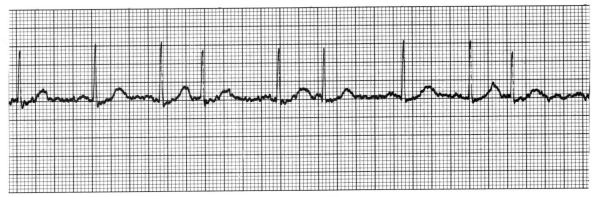

PRACTICE STRIP #14

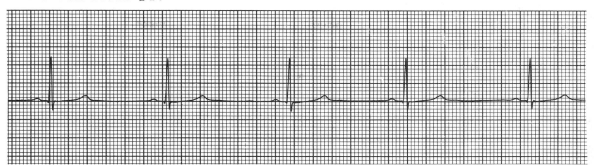

PRACTICE STRIP #15

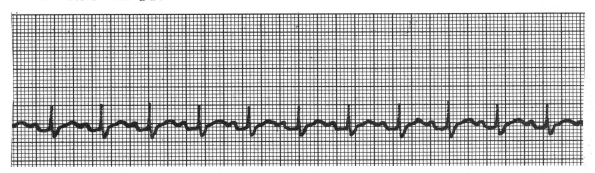

PRACTICE STRIP #16

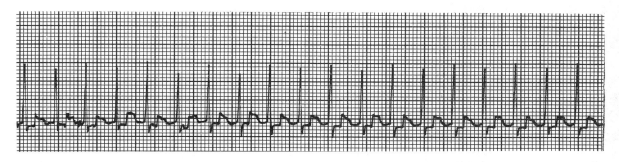

PRACTICE STRIP #17

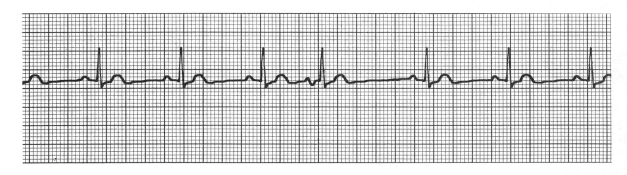

PRACTICE STRIP #18

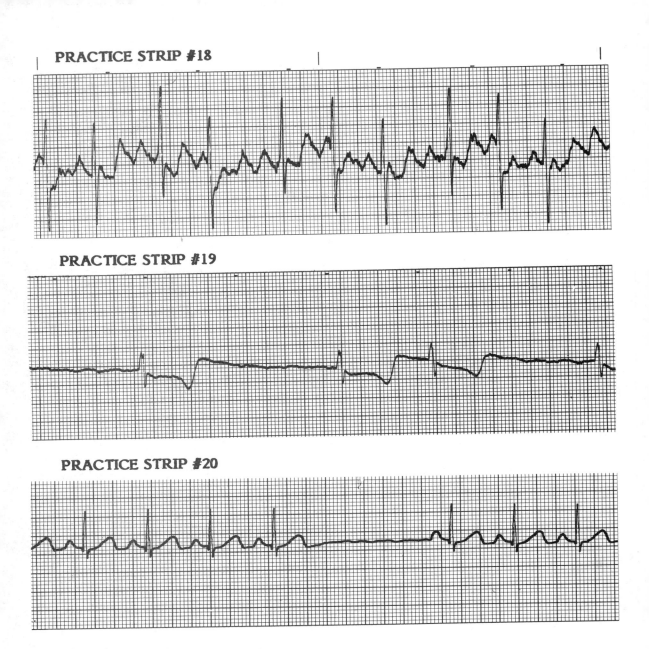

PRACTICE STRIP #19

PRACTICE STRIP #20

PRACTICE STRIP #21

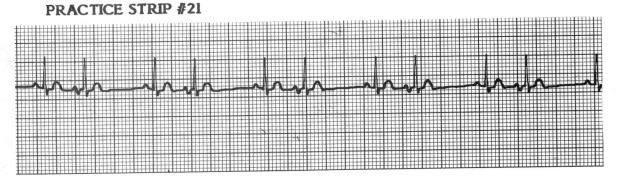

PRACTICE STRIP #22

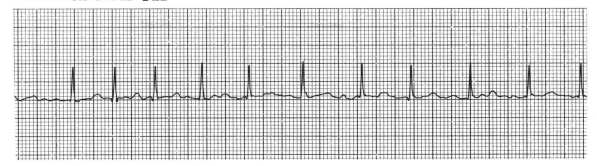

PRACTICE STRIP #23

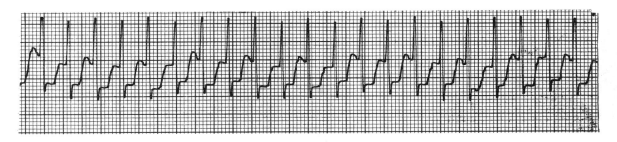

PRACTICE STRIP #24

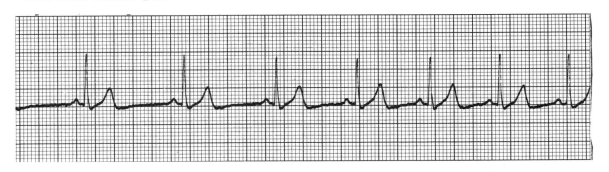

PRACTICE STRIP #25

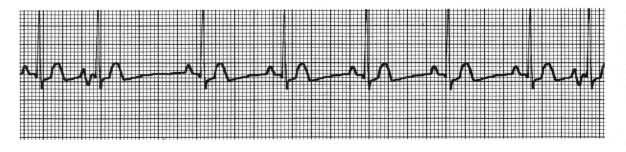

PRACTICE STRIP #26

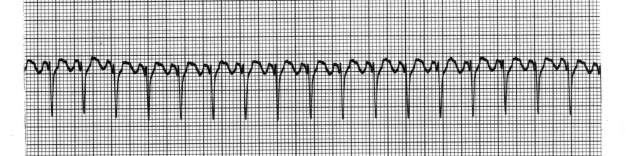

PRACTICE STRIP #27

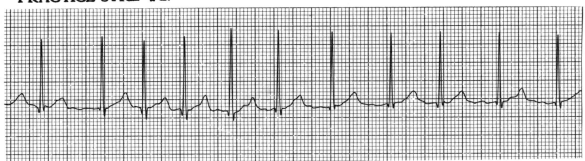

PRACTICE STRIP #28

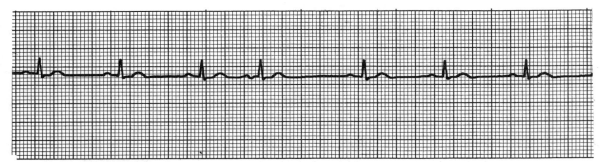

PRACTICE STRIP #29

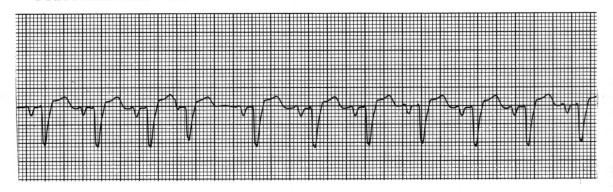

ANSWERS TO PRACTICE STRIPS

PRACTICE STRIP #10

Atrial Rhythm:	Regular
Ventricular Rhythm:	Regular
Atrial Rate:	90
Ventricular Rate:	90
P Waves:	P waves present, one P/complex, uniform
PRI:	.20 seconds
QRS:	.10 seconds
Interpretation:	Regular Sinus Rhythm (RSR)

PRACTICE STRIP #11

Atrial Rhythm:	Regular
Ventricular Rhythm:	Regular
Atrial Rate:	280
Ventricular Rate:	70
P Waves:	Flutter waves present
PRI:	Unable to measure
QRS:	.08 seconds
Interpretation:	Atrial Flutter 4:1

PRACTICE STRIP #12

Atrial Rhythm:	Unable to measure
Ventricular Rhythm:	Irregular
Atrial Rate:	Unable to measure
Ventricular Rate:	160
P Waves:	Unable to identify
PRI:	Unable to measure
QRS:	.06 seconds
Interpretation:	Atrial Fibrillation, Uncontrolled

ANSWERS TO PRACTICE STRIPS

PRACTICE STRIP #13

Atrial Rhythm:	Unable to measure
Ventricular Rhythm:	Irregular
Atrial Rate:	Unable to measure
Ventricular Rate:	90
P Waves:	Unable to identify
PRI:	Unable to measure
QRS:	.06 seconds
Interpretation:	Atrial Fibrillation, Controlled

PRACTICE STRIP #14

Atrial Rhythm:	Regular
Ventricular Rhythm:	Regular
Atrial Rate:	50
Ventricular Rate:	50
P Waves:	P waves present, one P/complex, uniform
PRI:	.16 seconds, constant
QRS:	.08 seconds
Interpretation:	Sinus Bradycardia

PRACTICE STRIP #15

Atrial Rhythm:	Regular
Ventricular Rhythm:	Regular
Atrial Rate:	190
Ventricular Rate:	190
P Waves:	P waves present, but difficult to see because the complexes are so close together
PRI:	Less than .20 seconds
QRS:	.08 seconds
Interpretation:	Atrial Tachycardia

ANSWERS TO PRACTICE STRIPS

PRACTICE STRIP #16

Atrial Rhythm:	Regular
Ventricular Rhythm:	Regular
Atrial Rate:	110
Ventricular Rate:	110
P Waves:	P waves present, one P/complex, uniform
PRI:	.20 seconds, constant
QRS:	.10 seconds
Interpretation:	Sinus Tachycardia

PRACTICE STRIP #17

Atrial Rhythm:	Regular except for the fourth beat
Ventricular Rhythm:	Regular except for the fourth beat
Atrial Rate:	70
Ventricular Rate:	70
P Waves:	P waves present, one P/complex, the fourth P is early and looks different than the others
PRI:	.16 seconds, constant
QRS:	.08 seconds
Interpretation:	Regular Sinus Rhythm (RSR) with one PAC

PRACTICE STRIP #18

Atrial Rhythm:	Regular
Ventricular Rhythm:	Irregular
Atrial Rate:	300
Ventricular Rate:	100
P Waves:	Flutter waves are present
PRI:	Unable to measure
QRS:	.10 seconds
Interpretation:	Atrial Flutter with Variable Conduction

ANSWERS TO PRACTICE STRIPS

PRACTICE STRIP #19

Atrial Rhythm:	Unable to measure
Ventricular Rhythm:	Irregular
Atrial Rate:	Unable to measure
Ventricular Rate:	40
P Waves:	Unable to identify
PRI:	Unable to measure
QRS:	.10 seconds
Interpretation:	Atrial Fibrillation with Bradycardia

PRACTICE STRIP #20

Atrial Rhythm:	Regular except for pause after the fourth beat
Ventricular Rhythm:	Regular except for pause after the fourth beat
Atrial Rate:	70
Ventricular Rate:	70
P Waves:	Present, one P/complex, no P wave during the pause
PRI:	.18 seconds, constant
QRS:	.08 seconds
Interpretation:	Regular Sinus Rhythm (RSR) with Sinus Arrest (or Sinus Pause which is a synonomous term)

PRACTICE STRIP #21

Atrial Rhythm:	Regularly Irregular
Ventricular Rhythm:	Regularly Irregular
Atrial Rate:	110
Ventricular Rate:	110
P Waves:	Present, one P/complex, every other one is early and looks different
PRI:	.12 seconds, constant
QRS:	.06 seconds
Interpretation:	Atrial Bigeminy with Tachycardia -- Every other beat is a PAC. When PAC's run in a pattern like this, i.e., one sinus to one PAC, it is called Atrial Bigeminy. PAC's can also run in a pattern of two sinus to one PAC--this is called Atrial Trigeminy. PAC's can also run in a pattern of three sinus to one PAC which is called Atrial Quadrigeminy!

ANSWERS TO PRACTICE STRIPS

PRACTICE STRIP #22

Atrial Rhythm:	Unable to measure
Ventricular Rhythm:	Irregular
Atrial Rate:	Unable to measure
Ventricular Rate:	110
P Waves:	Unable to identify
PRI:	Unable to measure
QRS:	.08 seconds
Interpretation:	Atrial Fibrillation, Uncontrolled

PRACTICE STRIP #23

Atrial Rhythm:	Regular
Ventricular Rhythm:	Regular
Atrial Rate:	210
Ventricular Rate:	210
P Waves:	P waves present, but difficult to see because the complexes are so close together
PRI:	Less than .20 seconds
QRS:	.08 seconds
Interpretation:	Atrial Tachycardia

PRACTICE STRIP #24

Atrial Rhythm:	Irregular
Ventricular Rhythm:	Irregular
Atrial Rate:	70
Ventricular Rate:	70
P Waves:	P waves present, one P/complex, uniform
PRI:	.14 seconds, constant
QRS:	.10 seconds, constant
Interpretation:	Sinus Arrhythmia

ANSWERS TO PRACTICE STRIPS

PRACTICE STRIP #25

Atrial Rhythm:	Regular except for the 2nd and 8th beat
Ventricular Rhythm:	Regular except for the 2nd and 8th beat
Atrial Rate:	80
Ventricular Rate:	80
P Waves:	P waves present; one P/complex, the 2nd and 8th P are early and look different than the others
PRI:	.16 seconds, constant
QRS:	.08 seconds
Interpretation:	RSR with 2 PAC's

PRACTICE STRIP #26

Atrial Rhythm:	Regular
Ventricular Rhythm:	Regular
Atrial Rate:	340
Ventricular Rate:	170
P Waves:	Flutter waves are present
PRI:	Unable to measure
QRS:	.08 seconds
Interpretation:	Atrial Flutter 2:1 (Every other Flutter Wave is interrupted on the ECG by a complex but it comes right back in on time.)

PRACTICE STRIP #27

Atrial Rhythm:	Unable to measure
Ventricular Rhythm:	Irregular
Atrial Rate:	Unable to measure
Ventricular Rate:	110
P Waves:	Unable to identify
PRI:	Unable to measure
QRS:	.08 seconds
Interpretation:	Atrial Fibrillation, Uncontrolled

ANSWERS TO PRACTICE STRIPS

PRACTICE STRIP #28

Atrial Rhythm:	Regular except for the 4th beat
Ventricular Rhythm:	Regular except for the 4th beat
Atrial Rate:	70
Ventricular Rate:	70
P Waves:	P waves present; one P/complex, the 4th P is early and looks different than the others
PRI:	.16 seconds, constant
QRS:	.06 seconds
Interpretation:	RSR with one PAC

PRACTICE STRIP #29

Atrial Rhythm:	Regular except for the 4th beat
Ventricular Rhythm:	Regular except for the 4th beat
Atrial Rate:	110
Ventricular Rate:	110
P Waves:	Biphasic P waves present; the 4th P (the P') is hiding in the previous T wave but you can find it if you look for it. Compare the 3rd T wave with the other T's on the strip. Notice the little point on it that is absent in the other T's! That is the P'! The Sinus waves here are biphasic which means that they are part above and part below the baseline. Biphasic P waves are normal in some leads.
PRI:	.20 seconds, constant
QRS:	.10 seconds (notice that the waves of the complex are QS and the elevated ST segment)
Interpretation:	Sinus Tachycardia with one PAC

CHAPTER 6: JUNCTIONAL ARRHYTHMIAS

The Junctional Arrhythmias originate from the A-V Junction.

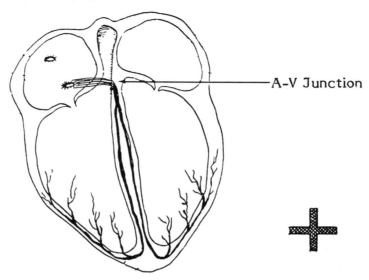

A-V Junction

To understand the Junctional Rhythms, you need to know that when depolarization moves towards a positive electrode, an upright wave is inscribed on the ECG and when depolarization moves away from a positive electrode, a negative wave is inscribed.

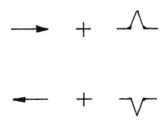

Most of the positive electrodes are on the left side of the chest and are depicted collectively as the large positive sign.

Since the A-V Junction is below the atria, depolarization of the atria will proceed from inferior to superior. This is called retrograde depolarization.

You can see that the atrial depolarization is moving away from the positive electrode.

QUESTION

What will be the configuration of the P wave when depolarization comes from the A-V Junction?

A. Right-side up (Positive P wave)
B. Upside down (Negative P wave)

ANSWER

B. The P wave will be a Negative deflection since atrial depolarization moves away from the positive electrode.

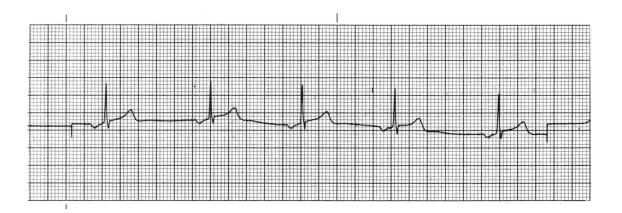

Notice the P wave in the above strip. It is a negative wave.

QUESTION

What is the PRI in the strip above?

ANSWER

.12 seconds

When you are able to measure PRI in the junctional ectopic arrhythmia, it will be .12 seconds or less. The A-V node does not delay retrograde conduction.

Depending on the speed of the retrograde conduction, atrial depolarization will occur before, after or at the same time as ventricular depolarization.

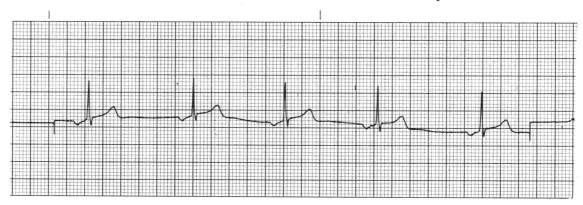

QUESTION

In the above strip, did atrial depolarization occur before, after or at the same time as ventricular depolarization?

ANSWER

Before. The P wave is inscribed before the complex.

When the atria and the ventricle depolarize together -- at the same time, we do not see a P wave because the atrial activity is lost on the ECG.

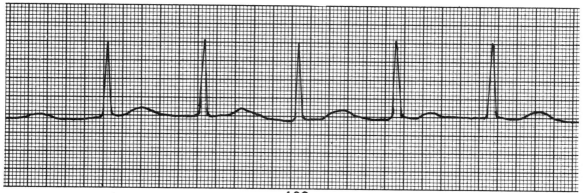

If the atria depolarizes <u>after</u> the ventricle, the P wave will be inscribed on the ECG; it will be after the complex and it will, of course, be upside down.

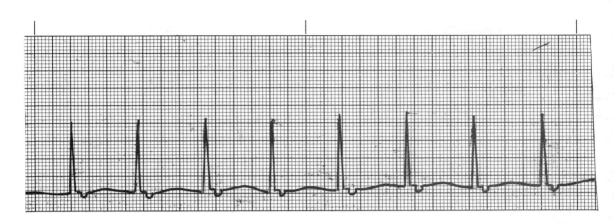

Depolarization of the atria is moving away from the positive electrode so we are going to see a negative P wave. However, in this case, depolarization reaches the ventricle FIRST (so you see the complex), then the atria depolarize and you see the negative P wave AFTER the complex!!!

In Review: You know the A-V Junction is the pacemaker if the P wave is either:

1. Negative before the complex with a PRI of .12 seconds or less.

2. Absent.

3. Negative after the complex.

There are six A-V Junctional Arrhythmias:

- Premature Junctional Contraction   - Junctional Escape Beat

- Junctional Tachycardia   - Junctional Escape Rhythm

     - Junctional Bradycardia

     - Accelerated Junctional Rhythm

PREMATURE JUNCTIONAL CONTRACTION (PJC)

PJC's, an irritable focus in the A-V Junction, depolarizes early.

The ECG characteristics of PJC are:

PREMATURE JUNCTIONAL CONTRACTION (PJC)

ATRIAL RHYTHM: Irregular due to the PJC

VENTRICULAR RHYTHM: Irregular due to the PJC

ATRIAL RATE: May be increased due to the PJC (Atrial activity will be lost in the complex if the atria and the ventricle depolarize at the same time.)

VENTRICULAR RATE: May be increased due to the PJC

P WAVE: P wave of the PJC is either inverted before or after the complex or it is absent.

PRI: .12 seconds or less if present

QRS: Less than .12 seconds

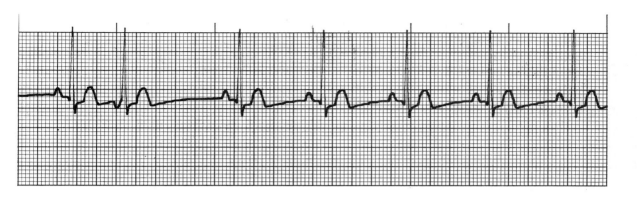

Using the above strip, fill in the following and check your answers with the correct answers in the right-hand column.

PRACTICE STRIP	ANSWERS
1. Atrial Rhythm: _____	1. Regular except for the 2nd beat
2. Ventricular Rhythm: _____	2. Regular except for the 2nd beat
3. Atrial Rate: _____	3. 70
4. Ventricular Rate: _____	4. 70
5. P Waves: _____	5. One P per complex; the P of the 2nd beat is inverted
6. PRI: _____	6. .16 seconds, PRI of 2nd beat is .10 seconds
7. QRS: _____	7. .10 seconds
8. Interpretation: _____	8. Regular Sinus Rhythm (RSR) with one PJC

If the A-V Junction is very irritable, it may usurp control and become the pacemaker of the heart.   This is called Junctional Tachycardia; it is an arrhythmia caused by an irritable focus in the A-V Junction.

The ECG Characteristrics of Junctional Tachycardia are:

JUNCTIONAL TACHYCARDIA

ATRIAL RHYTHM: Regular

VENTRICULAR RHYTHM: Regular

ATRIAL RATE: 101 to 200

VENTRICULAR RATE: 101 to 200

P WAVE: Either inverted before or after the complex or it is absent

PRI: .12 seconds or less if present

QRS: Less than .12 seconds

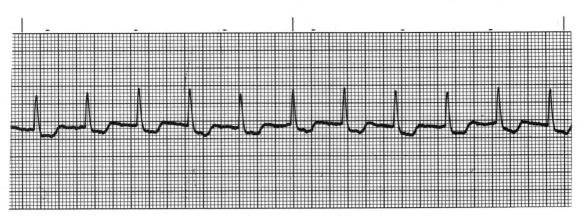

Using the above strip, fill in the following and check your answers with the correct answers in the right-hand column.

QUESTION	ANSWER
1. Atrial Rhythm: _____	1. Lost in the complex, must be Regular
2. Ventricular Rhythm: _____	2. Regular
3. Atrial Rate: _____	3. Lost in the complex
4. Ventricular Rate: _____	4. 110
5. P Waves: _____	5. Absent
6. PRI: _____	6. Unable to measure
7. QRS: _____	7. .06 seconds
8. Interpretation: _____	8. Junctional Tachycardia

JUNCTIONAL ESCAPE BEAT

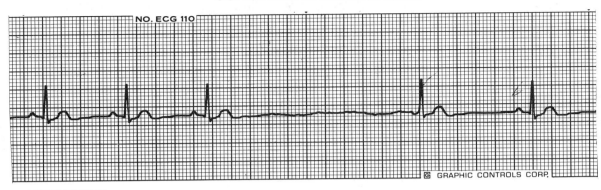

NO. ECG 110

Ⓖ GRAPHIC CONTROLS CORP.

QUESTION

On the above strip what happened to the sinus node?

ANSWER

The sinus Node arrested.

Notice the fourth complex. Where did it come from? You should be able to see there is no sinus P wave before that fourth complex. This complex originated from the A-V Junction. This is an escape beat. Escape beats occur because higher pacemakers have failed. Escape beats are life-saving mechanisms.

The ECG Characteristics of Junctional Escape Beats are:

JUNCTIONAL ESCAPE BEATS

ATRIAL RHYTHM:	Irregular due to the sinus arrest
VENTRICULAR RHYTHM:	Irregular due to the sinus arrest
ATRIAL RATE:	That of the underlying sinus rhythm; slowed due to the sinus arrest
VENTRICULAR RATE:	That of the underlying sinus rhythm; slowed due to the sinus arrest
P WAVE:	P wave of the Junctional Escape Beat will be inverted before or after the complex or it will be absent
PRI:	.12 seconds or less if present
QRS:	Less than .12 seconds

In the previous strip the sinus node "woke up" and took over as the pacemaker of the heart. Unfortunately, the sinus node does not always recover, in which case the A-V Junction can take over as pacemaker of the heart. This is a life-saving mechanism. The inherent firing rate of the A-V Junction is 40 to 60 times per minute.

The ECG Characteristics of Junctional Escape Rhythm are:

JUNCTIONAL ESCAPE RHYTHM

ATRIAL RHYTHM: Regular

VENTRICULAR RHYTHM: Regular

ATRIAL RATE: 40 to 60

VENTRICULAR RATE: 40 to 60

P WAVE: Inverted before or after the complex, or absent

PRI: .12 seconds or less when present

QRS: Less than .12 seconds

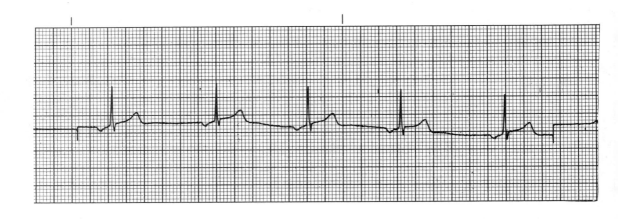

Using the above strip, fill in the following and check your answers with the correct answers in the right-hand column.

PRACTICE STRIP	ANSWERS
1. Atrial Rhythm: _____	1. Regular
2. Ventricular Rhythm: _____	2. Regular
3. Atrial Rate: _____	3. 50
4. Ventricular Rate: _____	4. 50
5. P Waves: _____	5. Present, one P/complex, inverted before the complex
6. PRI: _____	6. .12 seconds
7. QRS: _____	7. .08 seconds
8. Interpretation: _____	8. Junctional Escape Rhythm

The A-V Junction may escape as a pacemaker, at a rate slower than its inherent firing rate of 40 to 60 times per miniute. This is called Junctional Bradycardia.

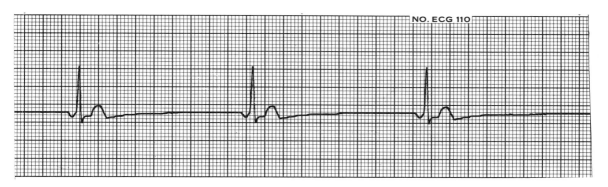

NO. ECG 110

Using the above strip, fill in the following and check your answers with the correct answers in the right-hand column.

PRACTICE STRIP	ANSWERS
1. Atrial Rhythm: _____	1. Regular
2. Ventricular Rhythm: _____	2. Regular
3. Atrial Rate: _____	3. $\emptyset$
4. Ventricular Rate: _____	4. 30
5. P Waves: _____	5. Present, inverted before the complex
6. PRI: _____	6. .08 seconds, constant
7. QRS: _____	7. .08 seconds
8. Interpretation: _____	8. Junctional Bradycardia

The A-V Junction may escape as a pacemaker, at a rate faster than its inherent firing rate of 40 to 60 times per minute but less than a tachycardia of 101. This is called Accelerated Junctional Rhythm.

The ECG Characteristics of Accelerated Junctional Rhythm are:

ACCELERATED JUNCTIONAL RHYTHM

ATRIAL RHYTHM: Regular

VENTRICULAR RHYTHM: Regular

ATRIAL RATE: 61 to 100

VENTRICULAR RATE: 61 to 100

P WAVE: Inverted before or after the complex or absent

PRI: .12 seconds or less when present

QRS: Less than .12 seconds

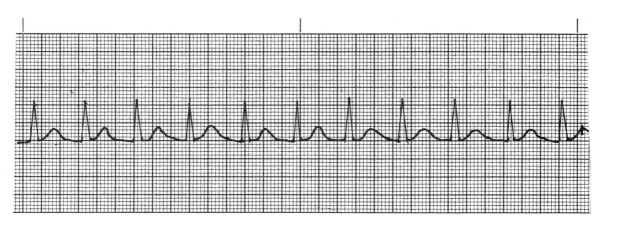

Using the above strip, fill in the following and check your answers with the correct answers in the right-hand column.

PRACTICE STRIP	ANSWERS
1. Atrial Rhythm: _____	1. Ø
2. Ventricular Rhythm: _____	2. Regular
3. Atrial Rate: _____	3. Ø
4. Ventricular Rate: _____	4. 110
5. P Waves: _____	5. Absent
6. PRI: _____	6. Ø
7. QRS: _____	7. .08 seconds
8. Interpretation: _____	8. Accelerated Junctional Rhythm

Accelerated junctional rhythms are relatively benign. Usually no treatment is required, provided the loss of atrial kick does not cause decreased cardiac output. If cardiac output is compromised, the sinus rate should be increased with atropine; if this fails, atrial pacing may be required.

In review the six junctional arrhythmias are:

-- Premature Junctional Contractions (PJC's)

-- Junctional Escape Beat

The sinus node is still the pacemaker of the heart. An irritable focus in the junction gives rise to a PJC. A temporary sinus arrest allows the junction to escape for a beat or two until the sinus recovers.

-- Junctional Bradycardia: less than 40

-- Junctional Escape Rhythm: 40-60

-- Accelerated Junctional Rhythm: 61-100

-- Junctional Tachycardia: 101-200

The Junction has taken over as the pacemaker of the heart.

You have learned the characteristics of the rhythms that originate in the sinus node and the atrial and junctional ectopic arrhythmias. On the following practice strips calculate the atrial and ventricular rates, the status of the P wave, the duration of the PRI and the ventricular complex. Then interpret the strip. You are reminded to make the measurements; do not just look at the answers. Refer to Chapter 9 page 266 to 273 for the causes, significance and appropriate interventions for the junctional arrhythmias.

The following practice strips consist of rhythms and arrhythmias originating from the sinus node, the atria and the A-V junction. Answers begin on page 123.

PRACTICE STRIP #30

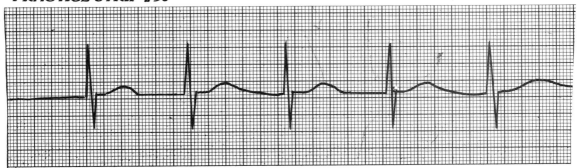

PRACTICE STRIP #31

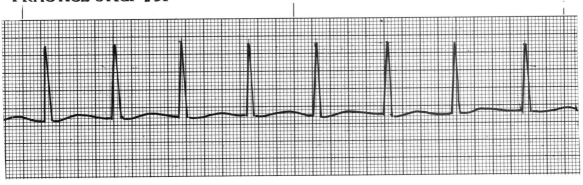

PRACTICE STRIP #32

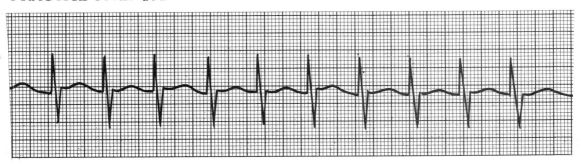

PRACTICE STRIP #33

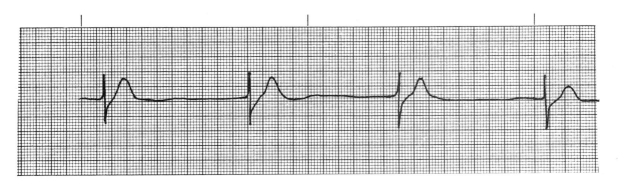

PRACTICE STRIP #34

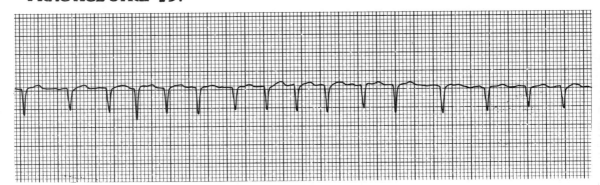

PRACTICE STRIP #35

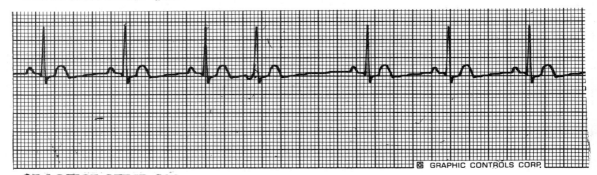

© GRAPHIC CONTROLS CORP.

PRACTICE STRIP #36

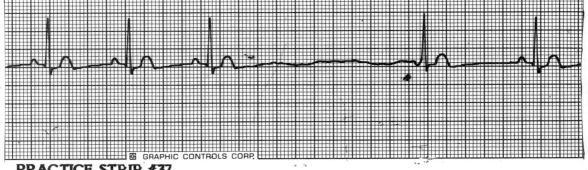

© GRAPHIC CONTROLS CORP.

PRACTICE STRIP #37

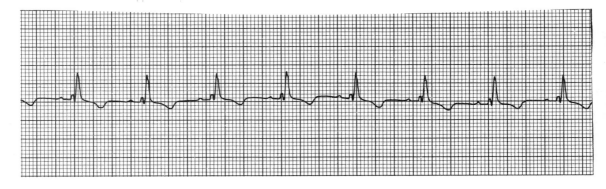

PRACTICE STRIP #38

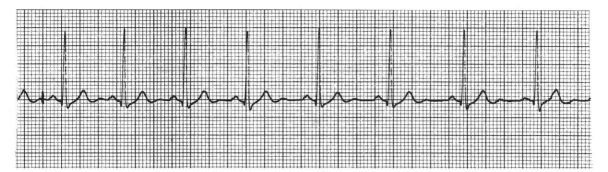

PRACTICE STRIP #39

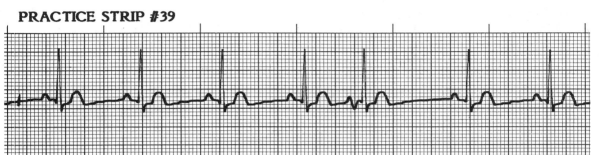

PRACTICE STRIP #40

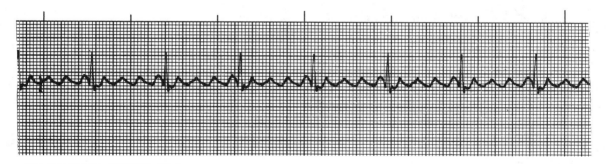

PRACTICE STRIP #41

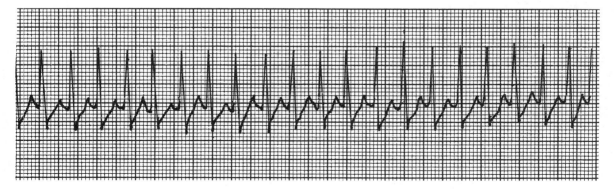

PRACTICE STRIP #42

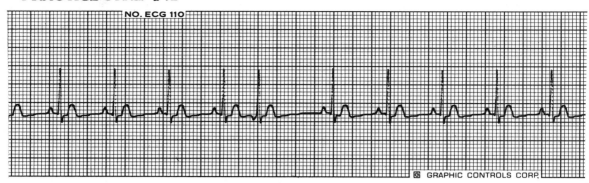

NO. ECG 110

G GRAPHIC CONTROLS CORP.

PRACTICE STRIP #43

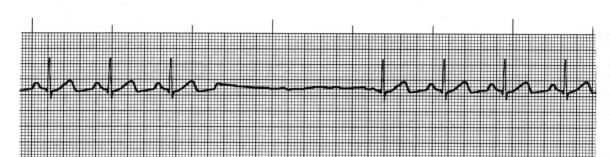

PRACTICE STRIP #44

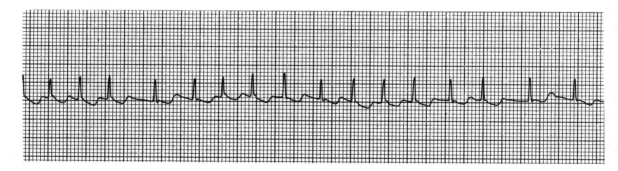

PRACTICE STRIP #45

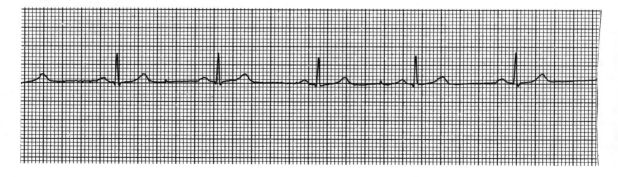

PRACTICE STRIP #46

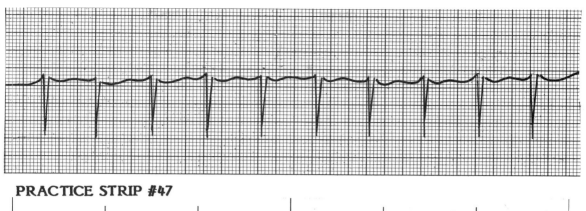

PRACTICE STRIP #47

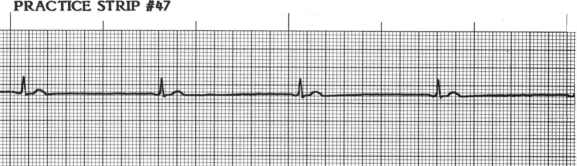

PRACTICE STRIP #48

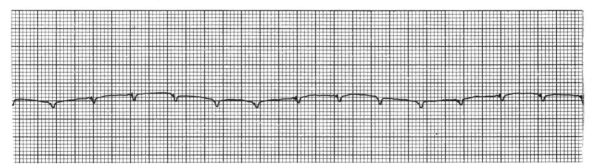

PRACTICE STRIP #49

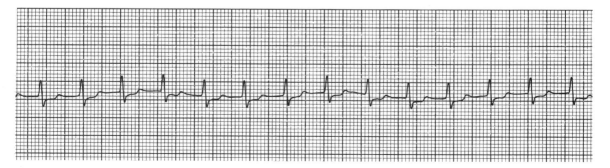

PRACTICE STRIP #50

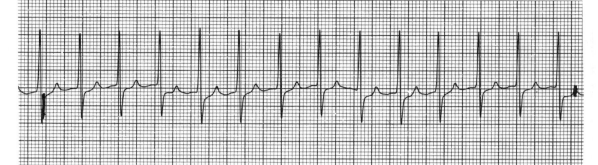

PRACTICE STRIP #51

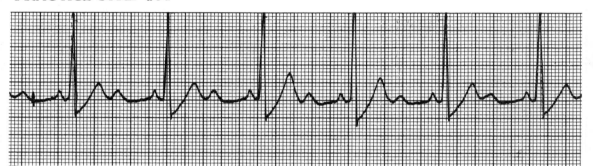

PRACTICE STRIP #52

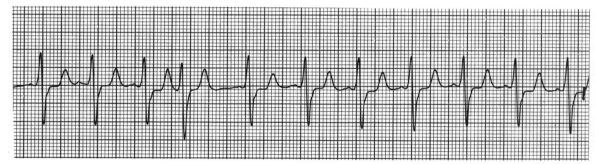

PRACTICE STRIP #53

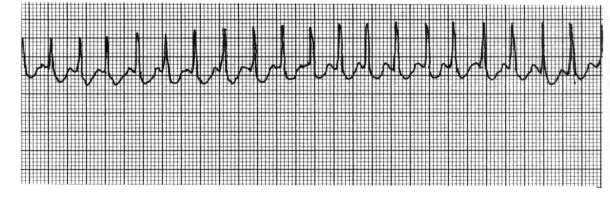

PRACTICE STRIP #54

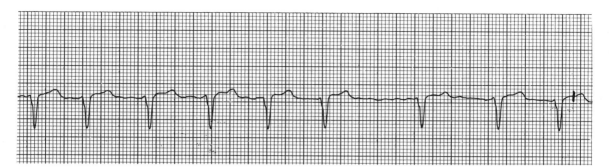

PRACTICE STRIP #55

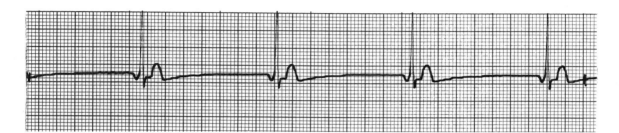

PRACTICE STRIP #56

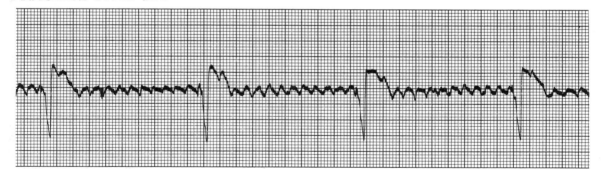

PRACTICE STRIP #57

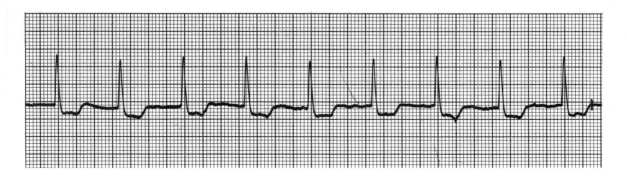

PRACTICE STRIP #58

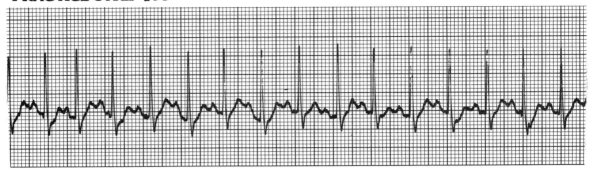

PRACTICE STRIP #59

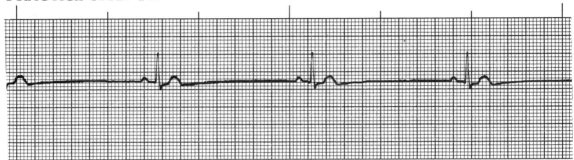

PRACTICE STRIP #60

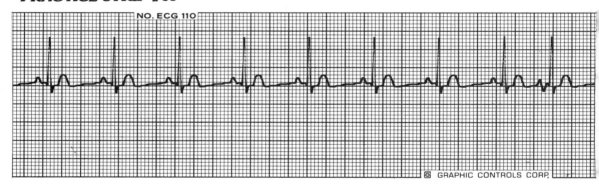

NO. ECG 110

Ⓖ GRAPHIC CONTROLS CORP.

ANSWERS TO PRACTICE STRIPS

PRACTICE STRIP #30

Atrial Rhythm:	Ø
Ventricular Rhythm:	Regular
Atrial Rate:	Ø
Ventricular Rate:	50
P Waves:	Absent
PRI:	Ø
QRS:	.10 seconds
Interpretation:	Junctional Escape Rhythm

PRACTICE STRIP #31

Atrial Rhythm:	Ø
Ventricular Rhythm:	Regular
Atrial Rate:	Ø
Ventricular Rate:	80
P Waves:	Ø
PRI:	Ø
QRS:	.08 seconds
Interpretation:	Accelerated Junctional Rhythm

PRACTICE STRIP #32

Atrial Rhythm:	Ø
Ventricular Rhythm:	Regular
Atrial Rate:	Ø
Ventricular Rate:	107 (Small Box Method)
P Waves:	Absent
PRI:	Ø
QRS:	.10 seconds
Interpretation:	Junctional Tachycardia

ANSWERS TO PRACTICE STRIPS

PRACTICE STRIP #33

Atrial Rhythm:	Ø
Ventricular Rhythm:	Regular
Atrial Rate:	Ø
Ventricular Rate:	30
P Waves:	Absent
PRI:	Ø
QRS:	.08 seconds
Interpretation:	Junctional Bradycardia

PRACTICE STRIP #34

Atrial Rhythm:	Unable to measure
Ventricular Rhythm:	Irregular
Atrial Rate:	Ø
Ventricular Rate:	160
P Waves:	Absent
PRI:	Unable to measure
QRS:	.04 seconds
Interpretation:	Atrial Fibrillation, Uncontolled (Did you interpret this Juctional Tachycardia? If so, you probably forgot that when the junction takes over as pacemaker it fires <u>regularly</u> and the ventricular rhythm is therefore <u>regular.</u>)

PRACTICE STRIP #35

Atrial Rhythm:	Regular except for the 4th beat
Ventricular Rhythm:	Regular except for the 4th beat
Atrial Rate:	70
Ventricular Rate:	70
P Waves:	Present except for the 4th beat; that beat is also early
PRI:	.16 seconds except for the 4th beat which is .08 seconds
QRS:	.08 seconds
Interpretation:	RSR with one PJC

ANSWERS TO PRACTICE STRIPS

PRACTICE STRIP #36

Atrial Rhythm:	Regular except for the arrest
Ventricular Rhythm:	Regular except for the arrest
Atrial Rate:	50 (underlying sinus rate is 75)
Ventricular Rate:	50
P Waves:	Present, one P per complex, uniform except for the escape beat (4th beat)
PRI:	.16 seconds except for the 4th beat which is .08
QRS:	seconds .08 seconds
Interpretation:	RSR with Sinus Arrest and Junctional Escape Beat (Sinus node regains control)

PRACTICE STRIP #37

Atrial Rhythm:	Regular
Ventricular Rhythm:	Regular
Atrial Rate:	80
Ventricular Rate:	80
P Waves:	Present, one P/complex, uniform
PRI:	.12 seconds, constant
QRS:	.12 seconds
Interpretation:	RSR with Aberrant Conduction to the Ventricles (Did you notice the rsR' configuration?)

PRACTICE STRIP #38

Atrial Rhythm:	Irregular
Ventricular Rhythm:	Irregular
Atrial Rate:	80
Ventricular Rate:	80
P Waves:	Present, one P/complex, uniform
PRI:	.16 seconds, constant
QRS:	.10 seconds
Interpretation:	Sinus Arrhythmia

ANSWERS TO PRACTICE STRIPS

PRACTICE STRIP #39

Atrial Rhythm:	Regular except for the 5th beat
Ventricular Rhythm:	Regular except for the 5th beat
Atrial Rate:	70
Ventricular Rate:	70
P Waves:	Present and uniform except for the 5th beat which is also early
PRI:	.16 seconds, constant
QRS:	.08 seconds
Interpretation:	RSR with one PAC

PRACTICE STRIP #40

Atrial Rhythm:	Regular
Ventricular Rhythm:	Regular
Atrial Rate:	300
Ventricular Rate:	70
P Waves:	Flutter waves are present
PRI:	Ø
QRS:	.08 seconds
Interpretation:	Atrial Flutter 4:1

PRACTICE STRIP #41

Atrial Rhythm:	Regular
Ventricular Rhythm:	Regular
Atrial Rate:	210
Ventricular Rate:	210
P Waves:	Present, but difficult to see because the complexes are so close together
PRI:	.12 seconds
QRS:	.08 seconds
Interpretation:	Atrial Tachycardia

ANSWERS TO PRACTICE STRIPS

PRACTICE STRIP #42

Atrial Rhythm:	Regular except for the 5th beat
Ventricular Rhythm:	Regular except for the 5th beat
Atrial Rate:	100
Ventricular Rate:	100
P Waves:	Present and uniform except for the 5th beat which is inverted before the complex
PRI:	.12 seconds, constant except for the 5th beat which is .06 seconds
QRS:	.06 seconds
Interpretation:	RSR with one PJC

PRACTICE STRIP #43

Atrial Rhythm:	Regular except for the pause
Ventricular Rhythm:	Regular except for the pause
Atrial Rate:	60 (4th P is lost in the complex)
Ventricular Rate:	60
P Waves:	Present and uniform except for the 4th beat which is late and does not have a P wave
PRI:	.18 seconds, constant
QRS:	.08 seconds
Interpretation:	RSR, Sinus Arrest, Junctional Escape Beat, RSR

PRACTICE STRIP #44

Atrial Rhythm:	Unable to measure
Ventricular Rhythm:	Irregular
Atrial Rate:	Unable to measure
Ventricular Rate:	160
P Waves:	Unable to identify
PRI:	Unable to measure
QRS:	.04 seconds
Interpretation:	Atrial Fibrillation, Uncontrolled

ANSWERS TO PRACTICE STRIPS

PRACTICE STRIP #45

Atrial Rhythm:	Regular
Ventricular Rhythm:	Regular
Atrial Rate:	50
Ventricular Rate:	50
P Waves:	P waves present, one P/complex, uniform
PRI:	.16 seconds, constant
QRS:	.06 seconds
Interpretation:	Sinus Bradycardia

PRACTICE STRIP #46

Atrial Rhythm:	Ø
Ventricular Rhythm:	Regular
Atrial Rate:	Ø
Ventricular Rate:	100
P Waves:	Ø
PRI:	Ø
QRS:	.06 seconds
Interpretation:	Accelerated Junctional Rhythm

PRACTICE STRIP #47

Atrial Rhythm:	Ø
Ventricular Rhythm:	Regular
Atrial Rate:	Ø
Ventricular Rate:	40
P Waves:	Ø
PRI:	Ø
QRS:	.06 seconds
Interpretation:	Junctional Escape Rhythm

ANSWERS TO PRACTICE STRIPS

PRACTICE STRIP #48

Atrial Rhythm:	Ø
Ventricular Rhythm:	Regular
Atrial Rate:	Ø
Ventricular Rate:	136 (Small Box Method/ 1500 ÷ 11 = 136)
P Waves:	Ø
PRI:	Ø
QRS:	.04 seconds
Interpretation:	Junctional Tachycardia (This was a difficult one-- difficult to see what is going on! See strip #49 & #50 below.)

PRACTICE STRIP #49

Atrial Rhythm:	Ø
Ventricular Rhythm:	Regular
Atrial Rate:	Ø
Ventricular Rate:	136 (Small Box Method)
P Waves:	Ø
PRI:	Ø
QRS:	.08 seconds
Interpretation:	Junctional Tachycardia (This tracing is from the same patient as #48 above. This is Lead II, #48 is Lead MCL1. If you can't see what's going on, change the lead to obtain a better picture.)

PRACTICE STRIP #50

Atrial Rhythm:	Ø
Ventricular Rhythm:	Regular
Atrial Rate:	Ø
Ventricular Rate:	140 (Six-Second Method)
P Waves:	Ø
PRI:	Ø
QRS:	.08 seconds
Interpretation:	Junctional Tachycardia (This is the same patient at the same time as #48 and #49 in still another lead. This lead is V5.)

ANSWERS TO PRACTICE STRIPS

PRACTICE STRIP #51

Atrial Rhythm:	Regular
Ventricular Rhythm:	Regular
Atrial Rate:	60
Ventricular Rate:	60
P Waves:	Present, one P/complex, uniform
PRI:	.12 seconds, constant
QRS:	.10 seconds
Interpretation:	RSR (Notice the large U wave and the depressed ST segment.)

PRACTICE STRIP #52

Atrial Rhythm:	Regular except for the 4th beat
Ventricular Rhythm:	Regular except for the 4th beat
Atrial Rate:	110
Ventricular Rate:	110
P Waves:	Present and uniform except preceeding the 4th beat which is also early
PRI:	.12 seconds, constant, except for the 4th beat
QRS:	.10 seconds
Interpretation:	Sinus Tachycardia with one PAC (One has to look very closely to find the P' of the PAC. Notice the 3rd T wave; it is pointed and one small box taller than the other T waves--that is the P'.)

PRACTICE STRIP #53

Atrial Rhythm:	Regular
Ventricular Rhythm:	Regular
Atrial Rate:	200
Ventricular Rate:	200
P Waves:	Present, difficult to see because the complexes are so close together
PRI:	.12 seconds, constant
QRS:	.04 seconds
Interpretation:	Atrial Tachycardia

ANSWERS TO PRACTICE STRIPS

PRACTICE STRIP #54

Atrial Rhythm:	Unable to measure
Ventricular Rhythm:	Irregular
Atrial Rate:	Unable to measure
Ventricular Rate:	90
P Waves:	Unable to identify
PRI:	Unable to measure
QRS:	.08 seconds
Interpretation:	Atrial Fibrillation, Controlled

PRACTICE STRIP #55

Atrial Rhythm:	Regular
Ventricular Rhythm:	Regular
Atrial Rate:	40
Ventricular Rate:	40
P Waves:	Present, inverted before the complex
PRI:	.08 seconds
QRS:	.06 seconds
Interpretation:	Junctional Escape Rhythm

PRACTICE STRIP #56

Atrial Rhythm:	Flutter pattern is present
Ventricular Rhythm:	Regular
Atrial Rate:	375
Ventricular Rate:	30
P Waves:	Flutter waves are present
PRI:	Ø
QRS:	.10 seconds
Interpretation:	Atrial Flutter with Bradycardia

ANSWERS TO PRACTICE STRIPS

PRACTICE STRIP #57

Atrial Rhythm:	Ø
Ventricular Rhythm:	Regular
Atrial Rate:	Ø
Ventricular Rate:	90
P Waves:	Ø
PRI:	Ø
QRS:	.08 seconds
Interpretation:	Accelerated Junctional Rhythm

PRACTICE STRIP #58

Atrial Rhythm:	Regular
Ventricular Rhythm:	Regular
Atrial Rate:	150
Ventricular Rate:	150
P Waves:	Present, one P/complex, uniform
PRI:	.16 seconds
QRS:	.08 seconds
Interpretation:	Sinus Tachycardia

PRACTICE STRIP #59

Atrial Rhythm:	Regular
Ventricular Rhythm:	Regular
Atrial Rate:	36 (Small Box Method)
Ventricular Rate:	36
P Waves:	Present, one P/complex, uniform
PRI:	.16 seconds, constant
QRS:	.06 seconds
Interpretation:	Sinus Bradycardia

ANSWERS TO PRACTICE STRIPS

PRACTICE STRIP #60

Atrial Rhythm:	Regular except for the last beat
Ventricular Rhythm:	Regular except for the last beat
Atrial Rate:	90
Ventricular Rate:	90
P Waves:	Present, one P/complex, uniform except for the last beat which is also early
PRI:	.12 seconds, constant
QRS:	.08 seconds
Interpretation:	RSR with one PAC

SUPRAVENTRICULAR TACHYCARDIA (SVT)

Sometimes it is impossible to tell the pacemaker site in a supraventricular tachycardia.

EXAMPLE:

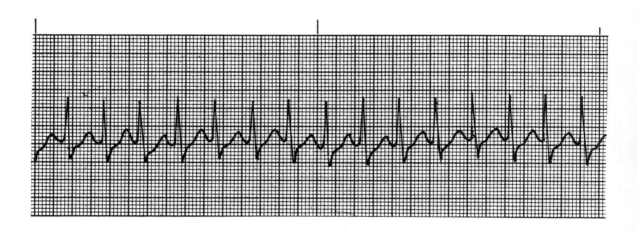

In the above strip, the rate is 150. It is impossible to say what is occurring between the complexes. Is that a T wave or a P wave, or is it a T with a P on top of it? If it is a T and there is no P, this would be Junctional Tachycardia. But if there is a P, the interpretation could be Sinus Tachycardia (rate 101 to 160) or Atrial Tachycardia (rate 150 to 250). We name this arrhythmia as best we can. We know the pacemaker is above the ventricles because the complex is less than .12 seconds -- so it is supraventricular; we know this is a tachycardia. Therefore, Supraventricular Tachycardia.

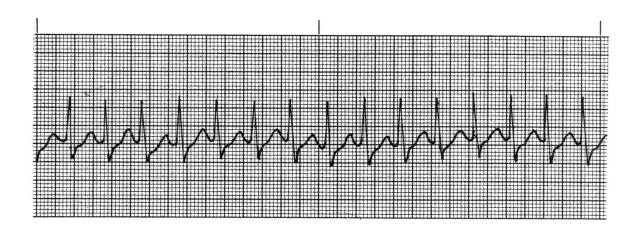

Using the above strip, fill in the following and check your answers with the correct answers in the right-hand column.

PRACTICE STRIP	ANSWERS
1. Atrial Rhythm: _____	1. Regular
2. Ventricular Rhythm: _____	2. Regular
3. Atrial Rate: _____	3. 150
4. Ventricular Rate: _____	4. 150
5. P Waves: _____	5. Unable to discern if there are P waves or not.
6. PRI: _____	6. Ø
7. QRS: _____	7. .10 seconds
8. Interpretation: _____	8. Supraventricular Tachycardia

WANDERING PACEMAKER

Sometimes the pacemaker site changes; the pacemaker may "wander" among the sinus node and atrial and junctional ectopics.   Although some beats originate from ectopic sites, the heart rate usually remains within a normal range.

EXAMPLE:

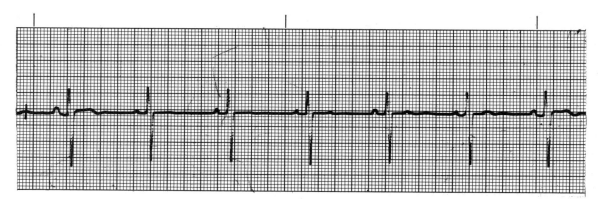

Note the changing contour of the P waves. The P's may also be inverted or missing when the pacemaker wanders into the A-V Junction.

The ECG characteristics of "wandering pacemakers" are three or more different configurations of the P wave in one lead. The PRI is less than .21 seconds. The rhythm is regular or may be slightly irregular.

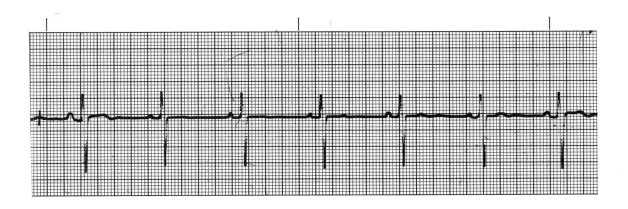

Using the above strip, fill in the following and check your answers with the correct answers in the right-hand column.

PRACTICE STRIP	ANSWERS
1. Atrial Rhythm: _____	1. Regular
2. Ventricular Rhythm: _____	2. Regular
3. Atrial Rate: _____	3. 60
4. Ventricular Rate: _____	4. 60
5. P Waves: _____	5. Present but not uniform
6. PRI: _____	6. .16 seconds, constant
7. QRS: _____	7. .08 seconds
8. Interpretation: _____	8. Wandering Pacemaker

CHAPTER 7: A-V HEART BLOCKS

A-V Heart Blocks occur because of pathology of the A-V node. When the A-V node is "sick" it is unable to do its job. The job of the A-V node is to conduct the impulse from the atria to the ventricle fast enough to result in a PRI of .12 to .20 seconds.

QUESTION

What is the normal PRI?

ANSWER

The normal PRI is .12 to .20 seconds

There are three degrees of A-V Heart Block but there are four categories of A-V Heart Block, as follows:

- First Degree A-V Heart Block

- Second Degree A-V Heart Block Type I (Mobitz I, Wenckebach)

- Second Degree A-V Heart Block Type II (Mobitz II)

- Third Degree A-V Heart Block (Complete Heart Block)

The "sicker" the A-V node, the higher the degree of block. First Degree and Second Degree Type I usually do not compromise the patient. Therefore, our intervention is just to observe the patient on the monitor. We observe to see if they develop a higher degree of block. Second Degree Type II and Third Degree are more dangerous and the definitive intervention is usually the insertion of an artificial pacemaker.

QUESTION

The intervention in First Degree and Mobitz I is to observe the patient on the monitor. What are you observing them for?

ANSWER

The development of a higher degree of block.

The ECG characteristics of First Degree A-V Heart Block are:

FIRST DEGREE A-V HEART BLOCK

ATRIAL RHYTHM: That of the prevailing rhythm

VENTRICULAR RHYTHM: That of the prevailing rhythm

ATRIAL RATE: 60 to 100 times per minute

VENTRICULAR RATE: 60 to 100 times per minute

P WAVE: Present and uniform; one P per complex

PRI: Greater than .20 seconds, constant

QRS: Less than .12 seconds

If you have First Degree A-V Heart Block with a rate greater than 100, the interpretation would be Sinus Tachycardia with First Degree A-V Heart Block.

If you have First Degree A-V Heart Block with a rate less than 60, the interpretation would be Sinus Bradycardia with First Degree A-V Heart Block.

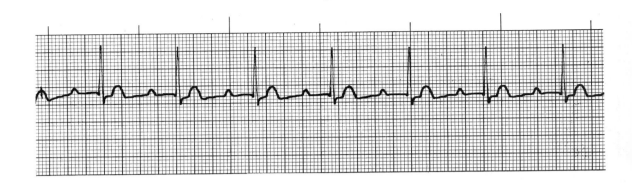

PRACTICE STRIP

Using the above strip, fill in the following and check your answers with the correct answers in the right-hand column.

QUESTION	ANSWER
1. Atrial Rhythm: _____	1. Regular
2. Ventricular Rhythm: _____	2. Regular
3. Atrial Rate: _____	3. 70
4. Ventricular Rate: _____	4. 70
5. P Waves: _____	5. Present & uniform; one P per complex
6. PRI: _____	6. .28 seconds, constant
7. QRS: _____	7. .08 seconds
8. Interpretation: _____	8. RSR with First Degree A-V Heart Block

CHAPTER 7:   A-V HEART BLOCKS (Cont'd)

There is a common characteristic between Second Degree A-V Heart Block Type I and Type II. This common characteristic is that there are more P's than complexes in both types.

Second Degree A-V Heart Block Type I is also called Mobitz I and Wenckebach.

The ECG characteristics of Second Degree A-V Heart Block Type I are:

SECOND DEGREE A-V HEART BLOCK TYPE I*

ATRIAL RHYTHM:	That of the prevailing rhythm
VENTRICULAR RHYTHM:	Irregular
ATRIAL RATE:	Usually normal
VENTRICULAR RATE:	Less than the Atrial Rate
P WAVE:	Present and uniform; more P's than complexes
PRI:	Progressively longer, until one P is blocked, then the cycle starts over again
QRS:	Less than .12 seconds

*Also called Wenckebach and Mobitz I

The secret of interpreting A-V heart blocks lies in the PRI. Second degree A-V Heart Block Type I, the PRI is variable, it is not constant. But there is a pattern to the variability, i.e., it gets longer and longer until a P does not conduct to the ventricles. Notice that the ventricular rhythm is irregular. It is "eyeball" irregular -- that is you do not have to measure with your calipers to see the ventricular irregularity. It is definitely irregular.

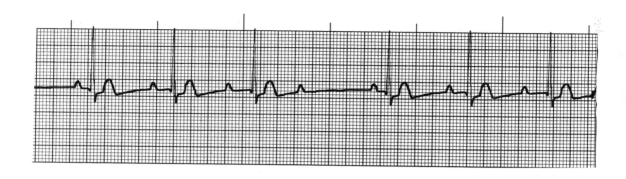

PRACTICE STRIP

Using the above strip, fill in the following and check your answers with the correct answers in the right-hand column.

QUESTION	ANSWER
1. Atrial Rhythm: _____	1. Regular
2. Ventricular Rhythm: _____	2. Irregular
3. Atrial Rate: _____	3. 70
4. Ventricular Rate: _____	4. 60
5. P Waves: _____	5. Present & uniform; more P's than complex
6. PRI: _____	6. Variable with a pattern that gets progressively longer until a P does not conduct; then the cycle starts over again.
7. QRS: _____	7. .08 seconds
8. Interpretation: _____	8. Second Degree A-V Heart Block Type I (Mobitz I, Wenckebach)

Second Degree A-V Heart Block Type II is also called Mobitz II. In this type of heart block, some P's conduct to the ventricle and some do not. The PRI of the P's that do conduct are constant.

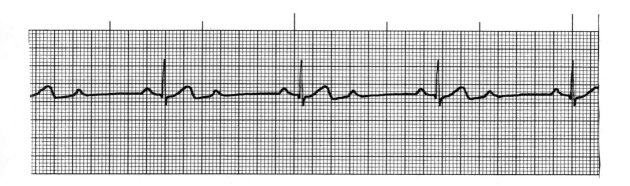

MOBITZ II

The PRI's in the above strip are all .20 seconds.

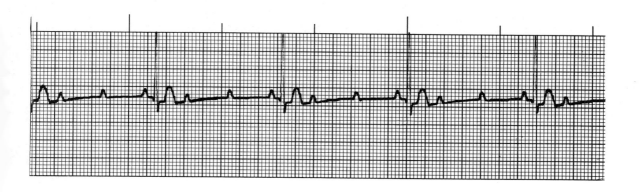

MOBITZ II

The PRI's in the above strip are all .12 seconds

The ECG characteristics of Second Degree A-V Heart Block Type II are:

SECOND DEGREE A-V HEART BLOCK TYPE II*

ATRIAL RHYTHM: That of the prevailing rhythm

VENTRICULAR RHYTHM: May be Regular or Irregular

ATRIAL RATE: That of the prevailing rhythm

VENTRICULAR RATE: Less than the Atrial Rate

P WAVE: Present; more P's than complexes

PRI: .12 seconds or greater. The PRI may be normal or prolonged; the PRI is constant for those P's that do conduct.

QRS: May be normal; however, a wide complex is not unusual and represents aberrant conduction through the ventricles.

*Also called Mobitz II

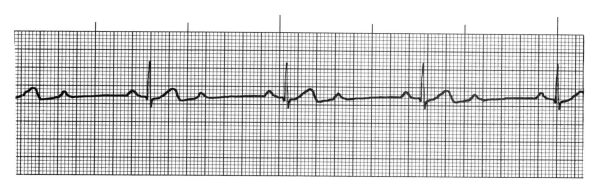

PRACTICE STRIP

Using the above strip, fill in the following and check your answers with the correct answers in the right-hand column.

QUESTION	ANSWER
1. Atrial Rhythm: _____	1. Regular
2. Ventricular Rhythm: _____	2. Regular
3. Atrial Rate: _____	3. 80
4. Ventricular Rate: _____	4. 40
5. P Waves: _____	5. Present & uniform; more P's than complex
6. PRI: _____	6. .20 seconds, constant for those P's that conduct
7. QRS: _____	7. .08 seconds
8. Interpretation: _____	8. Second Degree A-V Heart Block Type II (Mobitz II)

In Third Degree A-V Heart Block, the A-V node is not functioning. No impulses are conducted from the atria to the ventricles. Recall that anatomically between the atria and the ventricles there is connective tissue that forms the A-V valves. This connective tissue has no electrical properties.

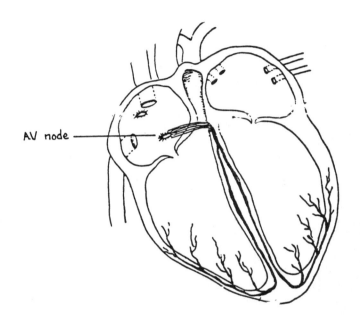

AV node

Electrical impulses in the atria must pass through the A-V node in order to get to the ventricles.

If the A-V node is not functioning, atrial electrical impulses cannot enter the ventricle. This is Third Degree A-V Heart Block. On the ECG, atrial electrical activity is unrelated to ventricular electrical activity; so you will see P waves totally unrelated to the complexes with a variable PRI. Since no impulse reaches the ventricle from the atria, a lower pacemaker will begin depolarizing the ventricle. This lower pacemaker may originate from the A-V junction or the ventricle itself. In Third Degree A-V Heart Block, there are two separate pacemakers pacing the heart; one pacing the atria inscribing P waves on the ECG, the other pacing the ventricles. These two pacemakers are totally unrelated to each other. This is a form of A-V dissociation.

CHAPTER 7: A-V HEART BLOCKS (Cont'd)

The ECG characteristics of Third Degree A-V Heart Block are:

THIRD DEGREE A-V HEART BLOCK

ATRIAL RHYTHM: That of the prevailing atrial rhythm

VENTRICULAR RHYTHM: Regular

ATRIAL RATE: That of the prevailing atrial rhythm

VENTRICULAR RATE: Slow

P WAVE: Present; unrelated to the complexes

PRI: Completely variable

QRS: Normal (less than .12 seconds), if the escape pacemaker originates from the A-V Junction. .12 seconds or greater if the escape pacemaker originates from the ventricle.

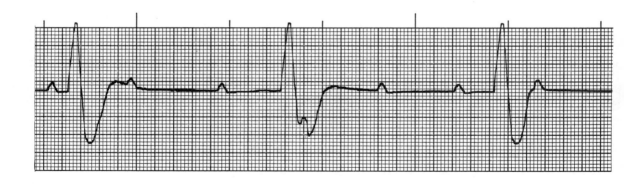

PRACTICE STRIP

Using the above strip, fill in the following and check your answers with the correct answers in the right-hand column.

QUESTION	ANSWER
1. Atrial Rhythm: _____	1. Regular
2. Ventricular Rhythm: _____	2. Regular
3. Atrial Rate: _____	3. 70 (counting the P that is in the ST segment in the second complex)
4. Ventricular Rate: _____	4. 30
5. P Waves: _____	5. Present unrelated to the complexes
6. PRI: _____	6. Variable without a pattern
7. QRS: _____	7. greater than .12 seconds
8. Interpretation: _____	8. Third Degree A-V Heart Block (Complete Heart Block)

Second Degree A-V Heart Block Type I (Mobitz I, Wenckebach) will sometimes masquerade as Complete Heart Block on the ECG. And, the opposite is true e.g., Complete Heart Block will masquerade as Second Degree A-V Heart Block Type I. This can lead to serious error in intervention. Recall the intervention for Mobitz I is observation, whereas the intervention for Complete Heart Block is the insertion of an artificial pacemaker! So, it is very important that you are not fooled.

HELPFUL HINT to differentiate Mobitz I from Complete Heart Block:

> In Mobitz I, the VENTRICULAR RHYTHM will be EYEBALL IRREGULAR. Eyeball irregular means you do not have to use your calipers to spot the irregular ventricular rhythm.

EXAMPLE

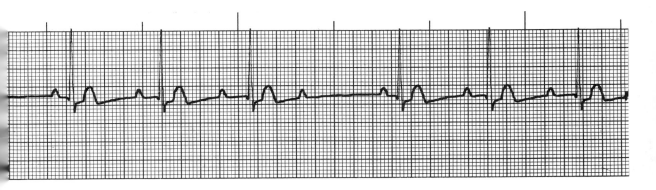

MOBITZ I

Notice the ventricular rhythm is "eyeball irregular."

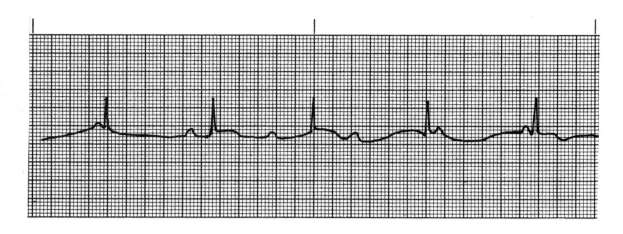

QUESTION

What is the interpretation of the above strip?

ANSWER

Complete Heart Block. Did you answer Mobitz I?

If you thought the above strip was Mobitz I, you did not learn the Helpful Hint that Mobitz I ventricular rhythm is <u>eyeball</u> <u>irregular</u>. Eyeball irregular means you can stand "across the room" and see that the ventricular rhythm is irregular. In the above strip the ventricular rhythm is caliper irregular; but it is NOT eyeball irregular.

Second Degree A-V Heart Block Type II (Mobitz II) will also masquerade as Complete Heart Block. And, the opposite is true, i.e. Complete Heart Block will masquerade as Mobitz II; but this is not too serious. Recall the definitive intervention for Mobitz II is the insertion of an artificial pacemaker and the definitive intervention for Complete Heart Block is also the insertion of an artificial pacemaker.

CHAPTER 7: A-V HEART BLOCKS (Cont'd)

Following is a summary of the A-V Heart Blocks. Remember, the A-V node is responsible for this group of arrhythmias. The A-V node controls the PRI. Therefore, the interpretation of A-V Heart Block rests in examining the PRI.

1° A-V HEART BLOCK

- Every P conducts
- PRI   greater than .20 seconds

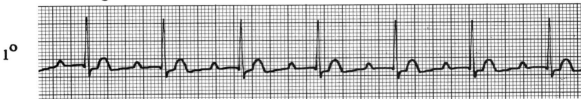

2° A-V HEART BLOCK TYPE I, MOBITZ I, WENCKEBACH

- More P's than complexes
- PRI progressively gets longer, until a P does not conduct--then the cycle starts over
- Ventricular rhythm "eyeball irregular"

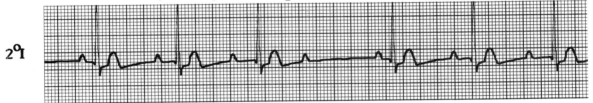

2° A-V HEART BLOCK TYPE II, MOBITZ II

- More P's than complexes
- PRI's constant and consistent

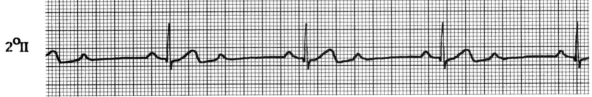

3° COMPLETE HEART BLOCK

- PRI variable (no P's are conducted)
- An escape pacemaker from the junction or the ventricle paces the ventricle

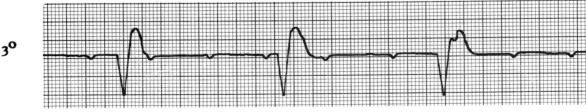

CHAPTER 7:   A-V HEART BLOCKS (Cont'd)

You have now learned the characteristics of the rhythms that originate in the sinus node, the atrial and junctional ectopic arrhythmias and the A-V Heart Blocks. On the following practice strips calculate the atrial and ventricular rate, the status of the P wave, the duration of the PRI and the ventricular complex. Then interpret the strip. You are again reminded to make the measurements and not to just look at the answers. Refer to Chapter 9 page 274 to 277 for the causes, significance and appropriate interventions for the A-V Heart Blocks. The following practice strips consist of rhythms and arrhythmias originating from the sinus node, the atria, the A-V junction and the A-V node. Answers began on page 161.

PRACTICE STRIP #61

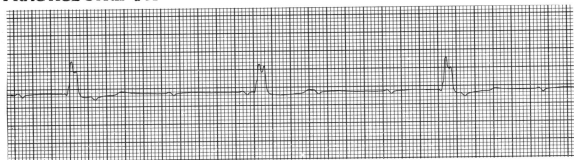

PRACTICE STRIP #62

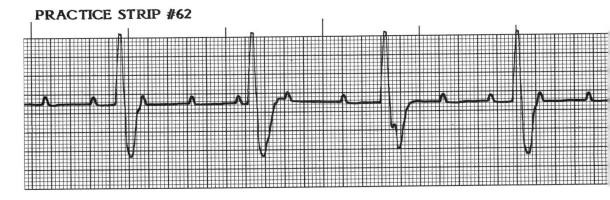

PRACTICE STRIP #63

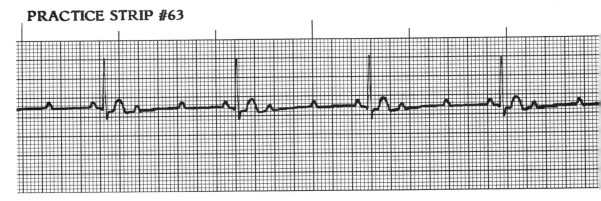

PRACTICE STRIP #64

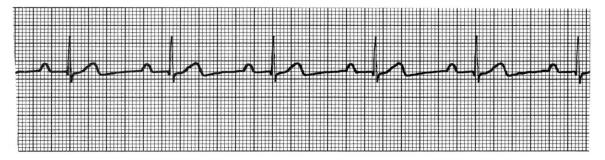

PRACTICE STRIP #65

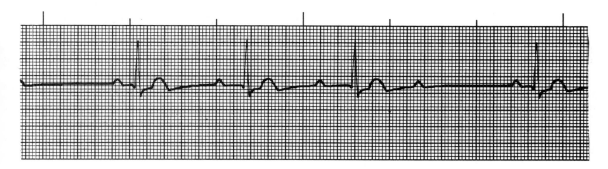

PRACTICE STRIP #66

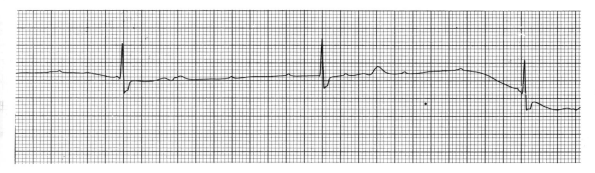

PRACTICE STRIP #67

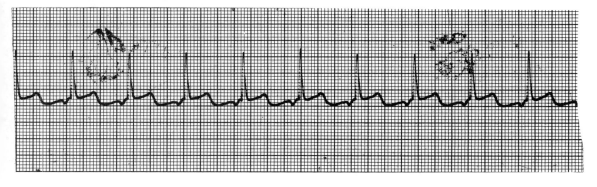

PRACTICE STRIP #68

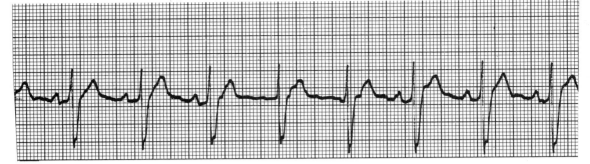

PRACTICE STRIP #69

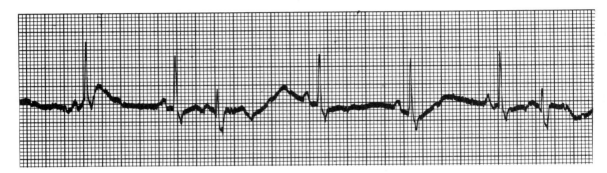

PRACTICE STRIP #70

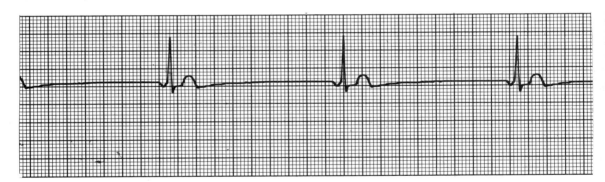

PRACTICE STRIP #71

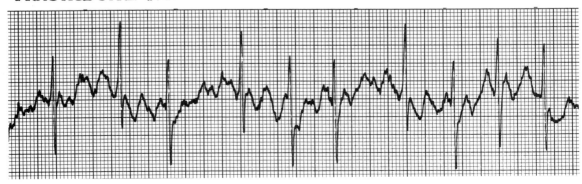

PRACTICE STRIP #72

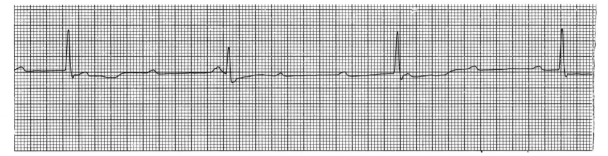

PRACTICE STRIP #73

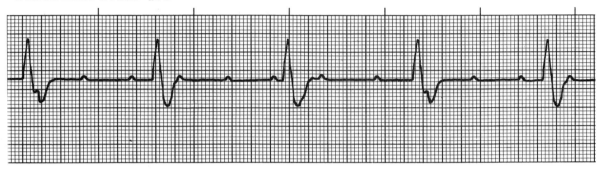

PRACTICE STRIP #74

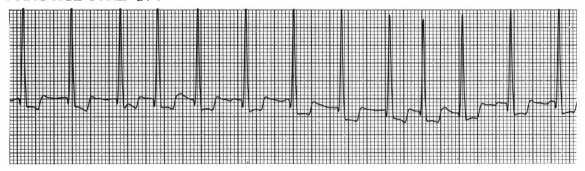

PRACTICE STRIP #75

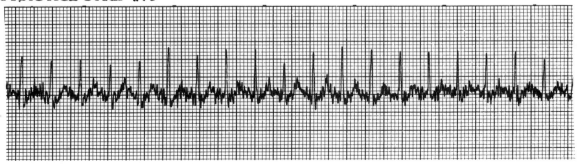

PRACTICE STRIP #76

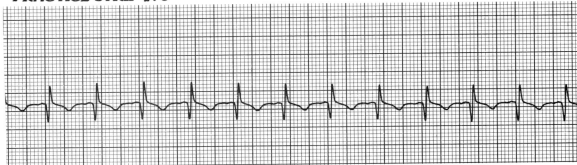

PRACTICE STRIP #77

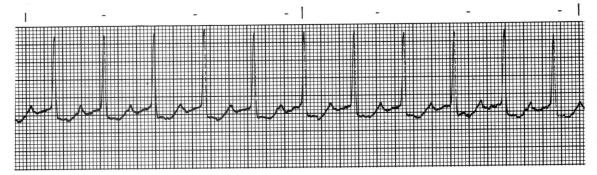

PRACTICE STRIP #78

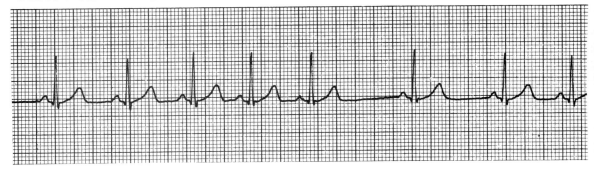

PRACTICE STRIP #79

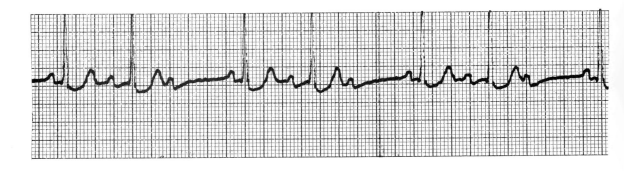

PRACTICE STRIP #80

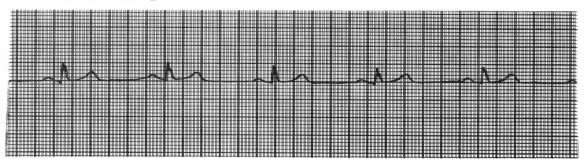

PRACTICE STRIP #81

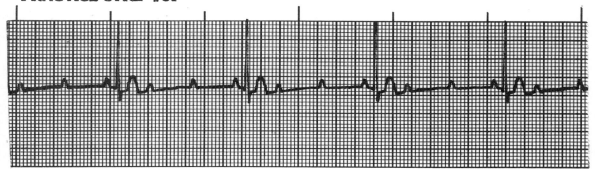

PRACTICE STRIP #82

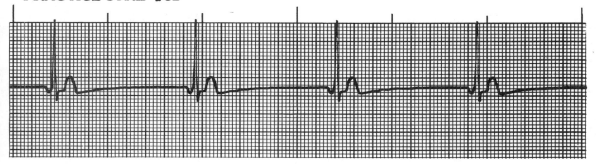

PRACTICE STRIP #83

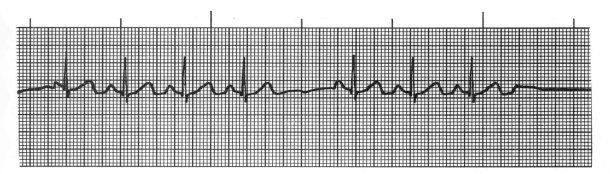

PRACTICE STRIP #84

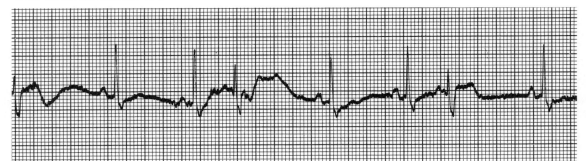

PRACTICE STRIP #85

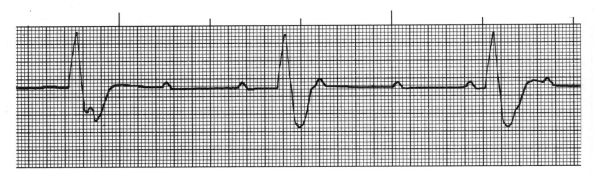

PRACTICE STRIP #86

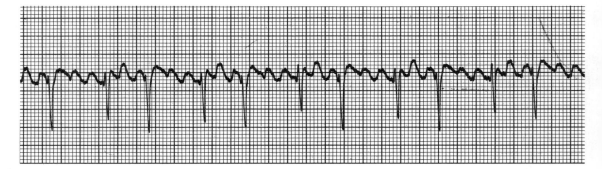

PRACTICE STRIP #87

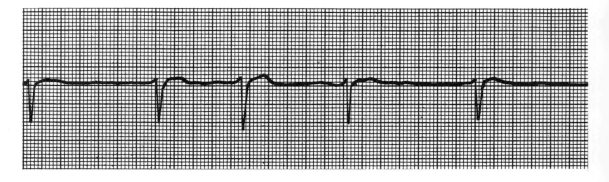

PRACTICE STRIP #88

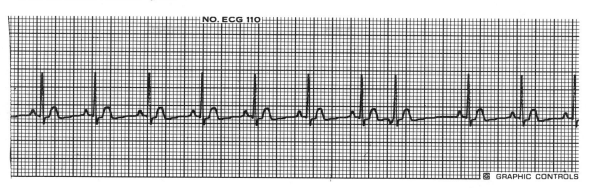

NO. ECG 110

GRAPHIC CONTROLS

PRACTICE STRIP #89

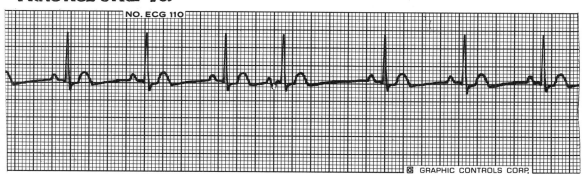

NO. ECG 110

GRAPHIC CONTROLS CORP.

PRACTICE STRIP #90

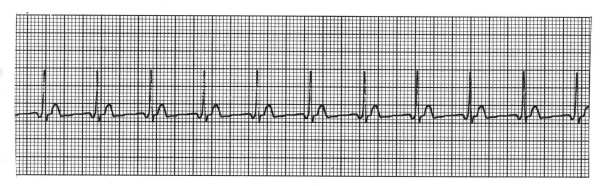

PRACTICE STRIP #91

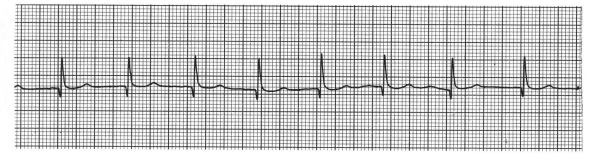

PRACTICE STRIP #92

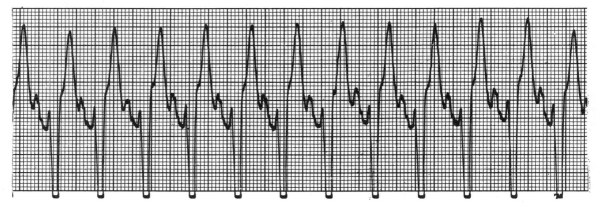

PRACTICE STRIP #93

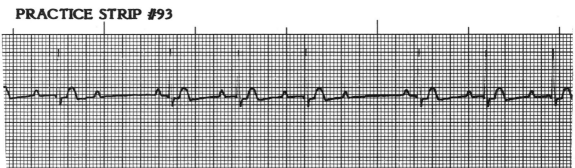

PRACTICE STRIP #94

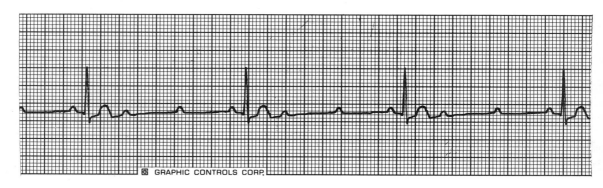

© GRAPHIC CONTROLS CORP.

PRACTICE STRIP #95

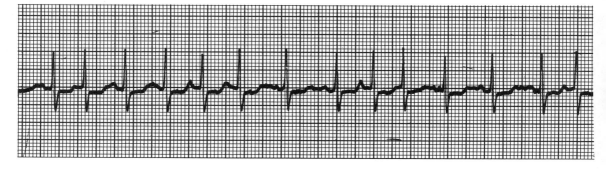

PRACTICE STRIP #96

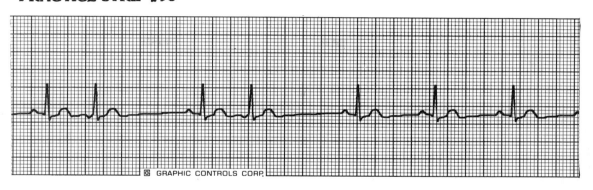

G GRAPHIC CONTROLS CORP.

ANSWERS TO PRACTICE STRIPS

PRACTICE STRIP #61

Atrial Rhythm:	Regular
Ventricular Rhythm:	Slightly irregular (not "eyeball irregular")
Atrial Rate:	80
Ventricular Rate:	30
P Waves:	Present, more P's than complexes
PRI:	Variable
QRS:	.10 seconds
Interpretation:	Third Degree A-V Heart Block (Complete Heart Block=CHB)

PRACTICE STRIP #62

Atrial Rhythm:	Regular
Ventricular Rhythm:	Regular
Atrial Rate:	120
Ventricular Rate:	40
P Waves:	Present, more P's than complexes
PRI:	Variable
QRS:	Greater than .12 seconds
Interpretation:	CHB

ANSWERS TO PRACTICE STRIPS

PRACTICE STRIP #63

Atrial Rhythm:	Regular
Ventricular Rhythm:	Regular
Atrial Rate:	130
Ventricular Rate:	40
P Waves:	Present, more P's than complexes
PRI:	.12 seconds, constant for those P's that conduct
QRS:	.06 seconds
Interpretation:	Second Degree A-V Heart Block Type II (Mobitz II)

PRACTICE STRIP #64

Atrial Rhythm:	Regular
Ventricular Rhythm:	Regular
Atrial Rate:	60
Ventricular Rate:	60
P Waves:	Present, one P/complex, uniform
PRI:	.28 seconds, constant
QRS:	.08 seconds
Interpretation:	RSR with First Degree A-V Heart Block

PRACTICE STRIP #65

Atrial Rhythm:	Regular
Ventricular Rhythm:	"Eyeball irregular"
Atrial Rate:	50
Ventricular Rate:	40
P Waves:	Present, more P's than complexes
PRI:	.24 to .40 seconds. Variable with a pattern; PRI becomes progressively longer until one P does not conduct.
QRS:	.10 seconds
Interpretation:	Second Degree A-V Heart Block Type I (Mobitz I) with Bradycardia

ANSWERS TO PRACTICE STRIPS

PRACTICE STRIP #66

Atrial Rhythm:	Slightly irregular
Ventricular Rhythm:	Regular
Atrial Rate:	100
Ventricular Rate:	30
P Waves:	Present, more P's than complexes
PRI:	Variable
QRS:	Greater than .12 seconds
Interpretation:	CHB (Complete Heart Block)

PRACTICE STRIP #67

Atrial Rhythm:	Regular
Ventricular Rhythm:	Regular
Atrial Rate:	90
Ventricular Rate:	90
P Waves:	Present, inverted before the complex, uniform
PRI:	.12 seconds
QRS:	.08 seconds
Interpretation:	Accelerated Junctional Rhythm

PRACTICE STRIP #68

Atrial Rhythm:	Regular
Ventricular Rhythm:	Regular
Atrial Rate:	80
Ventricular Rate:	80
P Waves:	Present, but not uniform
PRI:	.20 seconds except for the 4th and 5th beats
QRS:	.12 seconds
Interpretation:	Wandering Pacemaker with Aberrant Ventricular Conduction

ANSWERS TO PRACTICE STRIPS

PRACTICE STRIP #69

Atrial Rhythm:	Regular except for the 3rd and 7th beats
Ventricular Rhythm:	Regular except for the 3rd and 7th beats
Atrial Rate:	70
Ventricular Rate:	70
P Waves:	Present, one P/complex, uniform except for the 3rd and 7th beats
PRI:	.16 seconds, constant
QRS:	.10 seconds
Interpretation:	RSR with 2 PAC's Conducted Aberrantly

PRACTICE STRIP #70

Atrial Rhythm:	Regular
Ventricular Rhythm:	Regular
Atrial Rate:	30
Ventricular Rate:	30
P Waves:	Present, inverted before the complex
PRI:	.08 seconds
QRS:	.08 seconds
Interpretation:	Junctional Bradycardia

PRACTICE STRIP #71

Atrial Rhythm:	Flutter waves are present
Ventricular Rhythm:	Irregular
Atrial Rate:	280
Ventricular Rate:	100
P Waves:	Flutter waves
PRI:	0
QRS:	.08 seconds
Interpretation:	Atrial Flutter with Variable Conduction

ANSWERS TO PRACTICE STRIPS

PRACTICE STRIP #72

Atrial Rhythm:	Regular
Ventricular Rhythm:	Regular
Atrial Rate:	70
Ventricular Rate:	30
P Waves:	Present, more P's than complexes, some of the P's are lost in the complex and the T wave
PRI:	Variable
QRS:	.10 seconds
Interpretation:	CHB

PRACTICE STRIP #73

Atrial Rhythm:	Regular
Ventricular Rhythm:	Regular
Atrial Rate:	120
Ventricular Rate:	50
P Waves:	Present, more P's than complexes
PRI:	Variable
QRS:	.14 seconds
Interpretation:	CHB

PRACTICE STRIP #74

Atrial Rhythm:	Unable to identify a P wave
Ventricular Rhythm:	Irregular
Atrial Rate:	Ø
Ventricular Rate:	130
P Waves:	Ø
PRI:	Ø
QRS:	.08 seconds
Interpretation:	Atrial Fibrillation, Uncontrolled (For some reason Atrial Fibrillation is one of the most difficult arrhythmias for

ANSWERS TO PRACTICE STRIPS

PRACTICE STRIP #74 (Cont'd)

people to learn. Recall the ECG hallmarks of Atrial Fibrillation are (1) No definite P waves and (2) irregular ventricular rhythm. So as soon as you say:

Atrial Rhythm: Unable to see a definite P wave
Ventricular Rhythm: Irregular

you have the necessary ECG characteristics to interpret Atrial Fibrillation.)

PRACTICE STRIP #75

Atrial Rhythm:	Too much artifact to see a P wave
Ventricular Rhythm:	Regular
Atrial Rate:	Ø
Ventricular Rate:	190
P Waves:	Ø
PRI:	Ø
QRS:	.08 seconds
Interpretation:	SVT

PRACTICE STRIP #76

Atrial Rhythm:	Regular
Ventricular Rhythm:	Regular
Atrial Rate:	120
Ventricular Rate:	120
P Waves:	Very small inverted P wave before the complex
PRI:	.11 seconds
QRS:	.08 seconds
Interpretation:	Junctional Tachycardia

ANSWERS TO PRACTICE STRIPS

PRACTICE STRIP #77

Atrial Rhythm:	Regular
Ventricular Rhythm:	Regular
Atrial Rate:	110
Ventricular Rate:	110
P Waves:	Present, one P/complex, uniform
PRI:	.28 seconds, constant
QRS:	.08 seconds
Interpretation:	Sinus Tachycardia with First Degree A-V Heart Block

PRACTICE STRIP #78

Atrial Rhythm:	Irregular
Ventricular Rhythm:	Irregular
Atrial Rate:	80
Ventricular Rate:	80
P Waves:	Present, one P/complex, uniform
PRI:	.14 seconds, constant (there is a little electrical artifact on the 5th P wave)
QRS:	.08 seconds
Interpretation:	Sinus Arrhythmia

PRACTICE STRIP #79

Atrial Rhythm:	Regular
Ventricular Rhythm:	Irregular
Atrial Rate:	100
Ventricular Rate:	70
P Waves:	Present, more P's than complexes
PRI:	Variable with a pattern .16 to .24 seconds
QRS:	.10 seconds
Interpretation:	Mobitz I (Wenckebach)

ANSWERS TO PRACTICE STRIPS

PRACTICE STRIP #80

Atrial Rhythm:	Regular
Ventricular Rhythm:	Regular
Atrial Rate:	50
Ventricular Rate:	50
P Waves:	Present, one P/complex, uniform
PRI:	.18 seconds, constant
QRS:	.10 seconds
Interpretation:	Sinus Bradycardia

PRACTICE STRIP #81

Atrial Rhythm:	Regular
Ventricular Rhythm:	Regular
Atrial Rate:	140
Ventricular Rate:	40
P Waves:	Present, more P's than complexes, uniform
PRI:	.14 seconds
QRS:	.08 seconds
Interpretation:	Mobitz II

PRACTICE STRIP #82

Atrial Rhythm:	Regular
Ventricular Rhythm:	Regular
Atrial Rate:	40
Ventricular Rate:	40
P Waves:	Present, inverted before the complex, uniform
PRI:	.06 seconds
QRS:	.08 seconds
Interpretation:	Junctional Escape Rhythm

ANSWERS TO PRACTICE STRIPS

PRACTICE STRIP #83

Atrial Rhythm:	Regular except for the two pauses
Ventricular Rhythm:	Regular except for the two pauses
Atrial Rate:	70
Ventricular Rate:	70
P Waves:	Present, one P/complex, absent during the two pauses
PRI:	.20 seconds
QRS:	.08 seconds
Interpretation:	RSR with two episodes of Sinus Arrest

PRACTICE STRIP #84

Atrial Rhythm:	Every 3rd beat interrupts regularity
Ventricular Rhythm:	Every 3rd beat interrupts regularity
Atrial Rate:	70
Ventricular Rate:	70
P Waves:	Present, one P/complex, every 3rd P is early and looks different
PRI:	.16 seconds
QRS:	.10 seconds, every 3rd complex conducts aberrantly
Interpretation:	Atrial Trigeminy (Remember when there is a pattern of one PAC to two sinus beats it is called atrial trigeminy.)

PRACTICE STRIP #85

Atrial Rhythm:	Regular
Ventricular Rhythm:	Regular
Atrial Rate:	70
Ventricular Rate:	30
P Waves:	Present, more P's than complexes
PRI:	Variable
QRS:	.20 seconds
Interpretation:	CHB

ANSWERS TO PRACTICE STRIPS

PRACTICE STRIP #86

Atrial Rhythm:	Regular
Ventricular Rhythm:	Irregular
Atrial Rate:	340
Ventricular Rate:	110
P Waves:	Flutter waves
PRI:	∅
QRS:	.08 seconds
Interpretation:	Atrial Flutter with Tachycardia and Variable Conduction

PRACTICE STRIP #87

Atrial Rhythm:	∅
Ventricular Rhythm:	Irregular
Atrial Rate:	∅
Ventricular Rate:	50
P Waves:	∅
PRI:	∅
QRS:	.08 seconds
Interpretation:	Atrial Fibrillation with Bradycardia

PRACTICE STRIP #88

Atrial Rhythm:	Regular except for the 8th beat
Ventricular Rhythm:	Regular except for the 8th beat
Atrial Rate:	100
Ventricular Rate:	100
P Waves:	Present and uniform except for the 8th beat which has an inverted P wave and is early
PRI:	.12 seconds
QRS:	.06 seconds
Interpretation:	RSR with one PJC

ANSWERS TO PRACTICE STRIPS

PRACTICE STRIP #89

Atrial Rhythm:	Regular except for the 4th beat
Ventricular Rhythm:	Regular except for the 4th beat
Atrial Rate:	70
Ventricular Rate:	70
P Waves:	Present, one P/complex, uniform except for the 4th beat which is also early
PRI:	.16 seconds and constant
QRS:	.08 seconds
Interpretation:	RSR with one PAC

PRACTICE STRIP #90

Atrial Rhythm:	Regular
Ventricular Rhythm:	Regular
Atrial Rate:	110
Ventricular Rate:	110
P Waves:	Present, inverted before the complex
PRI:	.04 seconds
QRS:	.06 seconds
Interpretation:	Junctional Tachycardia

PRACTICE STRIP #91

Atrial Rhythm:	Ø
Ventricular Rhythm:	Regular
Atrial Rate:	Ø
Ventricular Rate:	80
P Waves:	Ø
PRI:	Ø
QRS:	.08 seconds
Interpretation:	Accelerated Junctional Rhythm

ANSWERS TO PRACTICE STRIPS

PRACTICE STRIP #92

Atrial Rhythm:	Regular
Ventricular Rhythm:	Regular
Atrial Rate:	120
Ventricular Rate:	120
P Waves:	Present, one P/complex, uniform
PRI:	.24 seconds, constant
QRS:	.12 seconds
Interpretation:	Sinus Tachycardia with First Degree A-V Heart Block, and Aberrant Ventricular Conduction

PRACTICE STRIP #93

Atrial Rhythm:	Regular
Ventricular Rhythm:	Irregular
Atrial Rate:	90
Ventricular Rate:	70
P Waves:	Present, more P's than complexes, uniform
PRI:	Variable .14 to .24 seconds
QRS:	.06 seconds
Interpretation:	Mobitz I

PRACTICE STRIP #94

Atrial Rhythm:	Regular
Ventricular Rhythm:	Regular
Atrial Rate:	100
Ventricular Rate:	40
P Waves:	Present, more P's than complexes, uniform
PRI:	.12 seconds, constant
QRS:	.08 seconds
Interpretation:	Mobitz II

ANSWERS TO PRACTICE STRIPS

PRACTICE STRIP #95

Atrial Rhythm:	Ø
Ventricular Rhythm:	Irregular
Atrial Rate:	Ø
Ventricular Rate:	140
P Waves:	Ø
PRI:	Ø
QRS:	.08 seconds
Interpretation:	Atrial Fibrillation, Uncontrolled (Because this is Course Atrial Fibrillation, every so often it looks like there may be a P wave. But there is no definite P wave. A definite P wave will be there every beat, not just every so often.)

PRACTICE STRIP #96

Atrial Rhythm:	Irregular due to the 2nd & 4th beats
Ventricular Rhythm:	Irregular due to the 2nd & 4th beats
Atrial Rate:	70
Ventricular Rate:	70
P Waves:	Present, inverted before the complex on the 2nd & 4th beats which are also early
PRI:	.14 seconds except for 2nd & 4th beats it is .08 seconds
QRS:	.06 seconds
Interpretation:	RSR with two PJC's

CHAPTER 8: VENTRICULAR ARRHYTHMIAS

The last pacemaker of the heart is the ventricle. Ventricular ectopic arrhythmias can be due to irritability or escape mechanisms. Since the ventricular ectopic originates in the ventricle, the impulse cannot travel the normal conduction system. Ventricular ectopics inscribe a wide complex on the ECG because it takes more time to depolarize the heart. The complex will be .12 seconds or longer in duration.

Abnormal depolarization is followed by abnormal repolarization; the ST-T segment is in a different direction than the main part of the complex.

If the complex is positive,

the ST-T will be negative

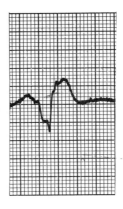

If the complex is negative,

the ST-T will be positive

Thus, ventricular ectopics appear wide and bizarre on the ECG.

PREMATURE VENTRICULAR CONTRACTIONS (PVC)

PVC's, an irritable forcus in the ventricle, depolarizes early.   The ECG characteristics of Premature Ventricular Contractions are:

PREMATURE VENTRICULAR CONTRACTIONS

ATRIAL RHYTHM: P wave is usually lost in the PVC

VENTRICULAR RHYTHM: The PVC will cause the rhythm to be irregular

ATRIAL RATE: The rate will be that of the underlying rhythm

VENTRICULAR RATE: The rate will be that of the underlying rhythm. PVC's may increase the ventricular rate.

P WAVE: Absent with the PVC's

PRI: Absent with the PVC's

QRS: .12 seconds or greater, wide and bizarre appearance

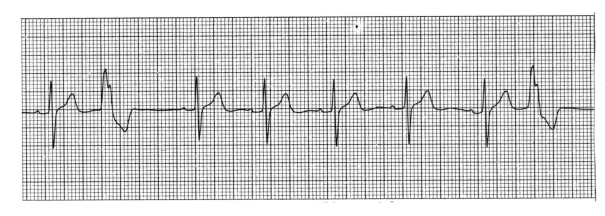

PRACTICE STRIP

Using the above strip, fill in the following and check your answers with the correct answers in the right-hand column.

QUESTION	ANSWER
1. Atrial Rhythm: _____	1. Regular except for 2nd & 8th beats
2. Ventricular Rhythm: _____	2. Regular except for 2nd & 8th beats
3. Atrial Rate: _____	3. 80 (2 P's hidden in 2nd & 8th complexes)
4. Ventricular Rate: _____	4. 80
5. P Waves: _____	5. Present & uniform; except for 2nd & 8th beats
6. PRI: _____	6. .16 seconds
7. QRS: _____	7. .08 seconds except for 2nd & 8th complexes which are greater than .12 seconds
8. Interpretation: _____	8. RSR with two PVC's

- Frequent PVC's are defined as six or more per minute. Frequent PVC's are usually treated.

- PVC's which are multifocal are more serious than unifocal PVC's:

EXAMPLE #1

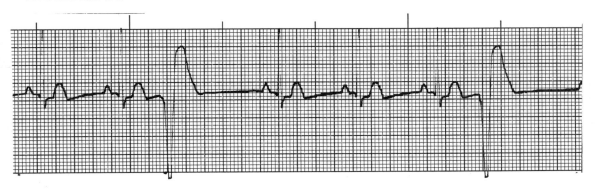

EXAMPLE #2

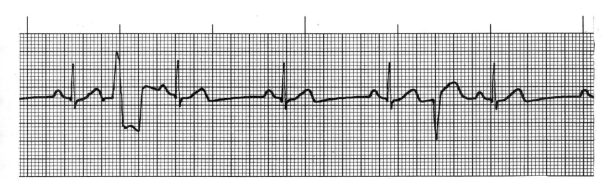

QUESTION:

Which of the above strips is an example of multifocal PVC's?

ANSWER

Example #2. The PVC's in Example #2 do not look alike. The fact that they look different on the ECG tells us that they depolarized the ventricle differently and therefore must have originated from different areas in the ventricle.

Two PVC's in a row are called sequential, or paired, or couplets.

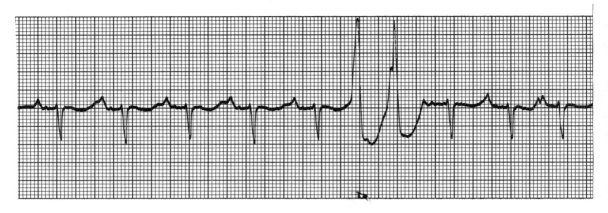

SEQUENTIAL PVC's

Three or more PVC's in a row is a run of Ventricular Tachycardia.

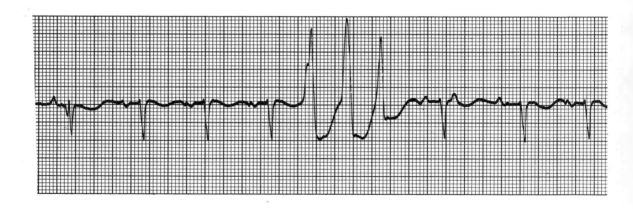

RUN OF VENTRICULAR TACHYCARDIA

Increasing frequency of PVC's is a warning of increasing ventricular irritibility and the possibility of progression to a more serious or even lethal ventricular arrhythmia.

PVC's also may occur in patterns like we saw with atrial and junctional prematures.

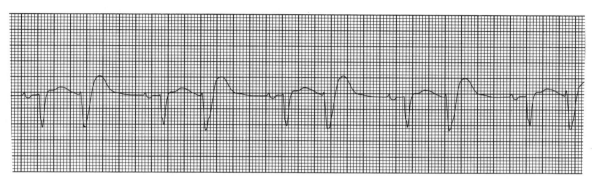

In the above strip there is one PVC with each sinus beat.

QUESTION:

What is the interpretation of the above strip?

ANSWER:

Ventricular Bigeminy.

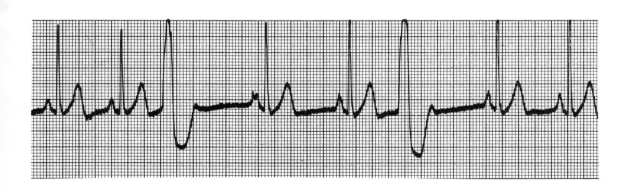

In the above strip, there is one PVC with every two sinus beats.

QUESTION:

How would you interpret the above strip?

ANSWER

Ventricular Trigeminy.

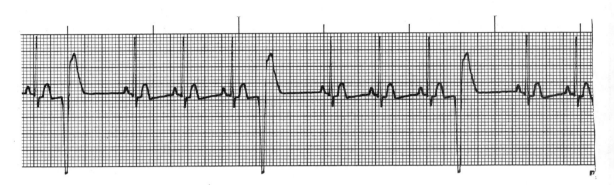

In the above strip there is one PVC with every three sinus beats.

QUESTION:

How would you interpret the above strip?

ANSWER

Ventricular Quadrigeminy.

In the previous examples of PVC's the sinus node regained control of the heart. If the ventricle is very irritible, it may usurp control and become the pacemaker of the heart. This is called Ventricular Tachycardia.

The ECG characteristics of Ventricular Tachycardia are:

VENTRICULAR TACHYCARDIA

ATRIAL RHYTHM: Usually not seen

VENTRICULAR RHYTHM: Usually Regular

ATRIAL RATE: Ø

VENTRICULAR RATE: 101 to 250

P WAVE: Usually lost in the complex but they may "peak through"

PRI: Ø

QRS: .12 seconds or greater. It is often difficult to tell the difference between the complex and its T wave as they merge together.

When Ventricular Tachycardia is faster than 250 times per minute, it is called Ventricular Flutter. Ventricular Tachycardia versus Ventricular Flutter is of academic importance only. With a ventricular rate of 250, the patient will have minimal, if any, cardiac output.

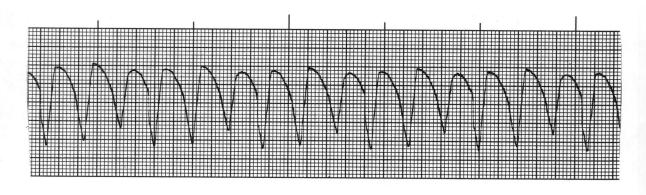

PRACTICE STRIP

Using the above strip, fill in the following and check your answers with the correct answers in the right-hand column.

QUESTION	ANSWER
1. Atrial Rhythm: _____	1. Ø
2. Ventricular Rhythm: _____	2. Regular
3. Atrial Rate: _____	3. Ø
4. Ventricular Rate: _____	4. 160
5. P Waves: _____	5. Ø
6. PRI: _____	6. Ø.
7. QRS: _____	7. .20 seconds, bizarre appearance
8. Interpretation: _____	8. Ventricular Tachycardia

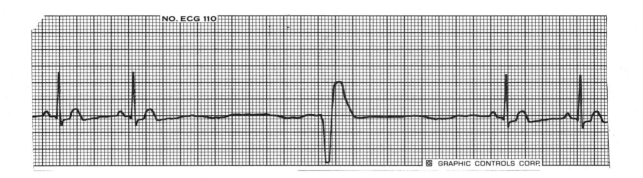

VENTRICULAR ESCAPE BEAT

On the above strip, notice the long pause after the second beat.

QUESTION

What happened to the sinus node?

ANSWER

The sinus node arrested.

Notice the third complex.   Where did it come from?   It is a ventricular ectopic -- a wide bizarre complex with the ST-T in the opposite direction to the main part of the complex.   This is a ventricular escape beat.   Escape beats occur because higher pacemakers have failed.   Escape beats are life-saving mechanisms.

On the above strip the sinus node "woke up" and took over as pacemaker of the heart.   Unfortunately, the sinus node does not always recover, in which case, the ventricle can take over as pacemaker of the heart.

The inherent firing rate of the ventricle is 15 to 40 times per minute.   When higher pacemakers fail, the ventricle is capable of pacing the heart.   This is called Idioventricular Rhythm when the ventricular pacemaker is firing 40 or less times per minute.

The ECG characteristics of Idioventricular Rhythm are:

IDIOVENTRICULAR RHYTHM

ATRIAL RHYTHM: Ø

VENTRICULAR RHYTHM: Usually Regular

ATRIAL RATE: Ø

VENTRICULAR RATE: Less than 40

P WAVE: Usually absent; if present they are not related to
                            the complex.
PRI: Ø
QRS: .12 seconds or more; wide and bizarre
                            appearance

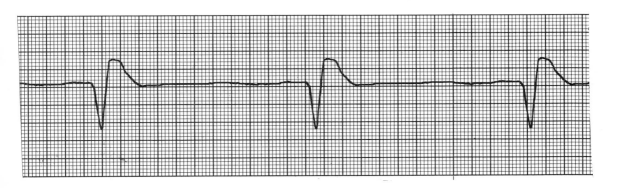

PRACTICE STRIP

Using the above strip, fill in the following and check your answers with the correct answers in the right-hand column.

QUESTION	ANSWER
1. Atrial Rhythm: _____	1. Ø
2. Ventricular Rhythm: _____	2. Regular
3. Atrial Rate: _____	3. Ø
4. Ventricular Rate: _____	4. 30
5. P Waves: _____	5. Ø
6. PRI: _____	6. Ø.
7. QRS: _____	7. .14 seconds, ST-T in opposite direction to the main part of complex
8. Interpretation: _____	8. Idioventricular Rhythm

The ventricle may escape as the pacemaker at a rate faster than its inherent firing rate of 15 to 40 times per minute but less than a tachycardia of 100. This is called Accelerated Ventricular Rhythm.

The ECG characteristics of Accelerated Ventricular Rhythm are:

ACCELERATED VENTRICULAR RHYTHM

ATRIAL RHYTHM: Ø

VENTRICULAR RHYTHM: Regular

ATRIAL RATE: Ø

VENTRICULAR RATE: 61 to 100

P WAVE: Ø

PRI: Ø

QRS: .12 seconds or greater

These accelerated ventricular rhythms may be relatively benign and usually do not require treatment. If cardiac output is decreased, the rate of the sinus node may be increased with atropine; if this fails, atrial pacing may be required.

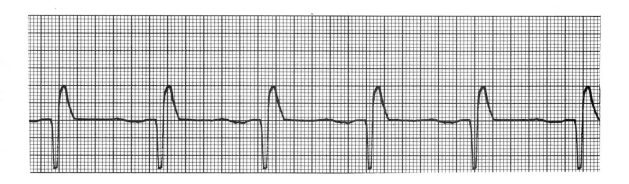

PRACTICE STRIP

Using the above strip, fill in the following and check your answers with the correct answers in the right-hand column.

QUESTION	ANSWER
1. Atrial Rhythm: _____	1. Ø
2. Ventricular Rhythm: _____	2. Regular
3. Atrial Rate: _____	3. Ø
4. Ventricular Rate: _____	4. 60
5. P Waves: _____	5. Ø
6. PRI: _____	6. Ø.
7. QRS: _____	7. .12 seconds, bizarre configuration
8. Interpretation: _____	8. Accelerated Ventricular Rhythm

The ECG characteristics of Ventricular Fibrillation are:

VENTRICULAR FIBRILLATION

ATRIAL RHYTHM: Totally chaotic rhythm

VENTRICULAR RHYTHM: Totally chaotic rhythm

ATRIAL RATE: Ø

VENTRICULAR RATE: Ø

P WAVE: Ø

PRI: Ø

QRS: No discernible QRS pattern.   Totally chaotic pattern on the ECG

In Ventricular Fibrillation, multiple foci in the ventricles become irritable and cause uncoordinated, chaotic impulses. The heart fibrillates; it does not contract. There is no cardiac output. The patient is clinically dead.

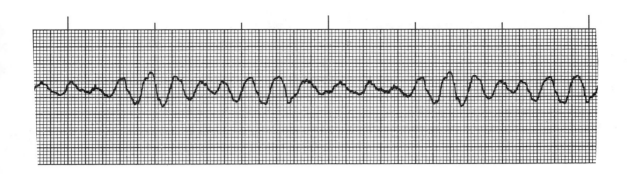

PRACTICE STRIP

Using the above strip, fill in the following and check your answers with the correct answers in the right-hand column.

QUESTION	ANSWER
1. Atrial Rhythm: _____	1. Totally chaotic rhythm
2. Ventricular Rhythm: _____	2. Totally chaotic rhythm
3. Atrial Rate: _____	3. 0
4. Ventricular Rate: _____	4. 0
5. P Waves: _____	5. 0
6. PRI: _____	6. 0.
7. QRS: _____	7. 0
8. Interpretation: _____	8. Ventricular Fibrillation

When the heart has lost its electrical activity there is a straight line recorded on the ECG. This is called Asystole.

The ECG characteristics of Asystole are:

ASYSTOLE

ATRIAL RHYTHM: No electrical activity is recorded; there is only a straight line on the ECG.

VENTRICULAR RHYTHM: No electrical activity is recorded; there is only a straight line on the ECG.

ATRIAL RATE: No electrical activity is recorded; there is only a straight line on the ECG.

VENTRICULAR RATE: No electrical activity is recorded; there is only a straight line on the ECG.

P WAVE: No electrical activity is recorded; there is only a straight line on the ECG.

PRI: No electrical activity is recorded; there is only a straight line on the ECG.

QRS: No electrical activity is recorded; there is only a straight line on the ECG.

PRACTICE STRIP

Using the above strip, fill in the following and check your answers with the correct answers in the right-hand column.

QUESTION	ANSWER
1. Atrial Rhythm: _____	1. Ø
2. Ventricular Rhythm: _____	2. Ø
3. Atrial Rate: _____	3. Ø
4. Ventricular Rate: _____	4. Ø
5. P Waves: _____	5. Ø
6. PRI: _____	6. Ø.
7. QRS: _____	7. Ø
8. Interpretation: _____	8. Asystole

You have now learned the characteristics of the rhythms that originate in the sinus node, the atrial, junctional and ventricular ectopic arrhythmias and the A-V Heart Blocks. On the following practice strips calculate the atrial and ventricular rates, the status of the P wave, the duration of the PRI and the ventricular complex. Then interpret the strip. You are reminded to make the measurements and not just look at the answers. Refer to Chapter 9 page 278 to 284 for the causes, significance and appropriate interventions for the ventricular arrhythmias.

The following practice strips consist of rhythms and arrhythmias originating from the sinus node, the atria, the A-V junction, the A-V node and ventricular ectopics. Answers begin on page 218.

PRACTICE STRIP #97

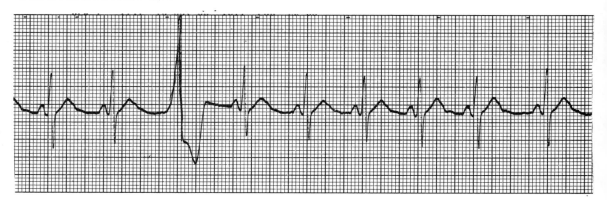

PRACTICE STRIP #98

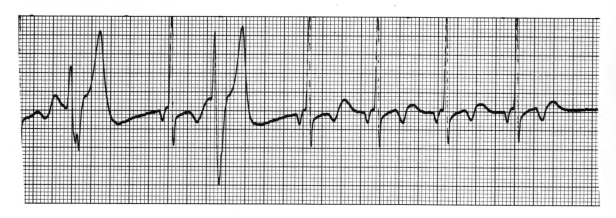

PRACTICE STRIP #99

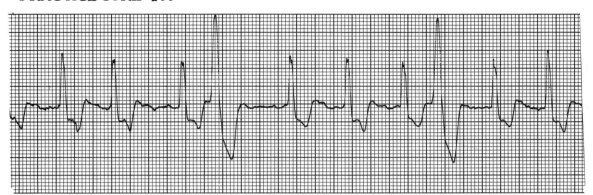

PRACTICE STRIP #100

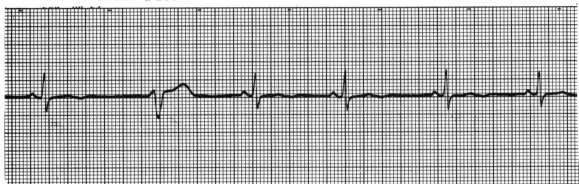

PRACTICE STRIP #101

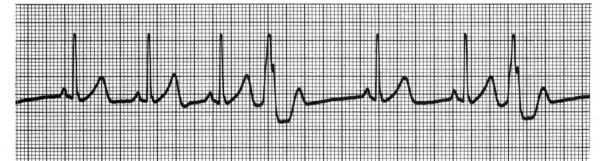

PRACTICE STRIP #102

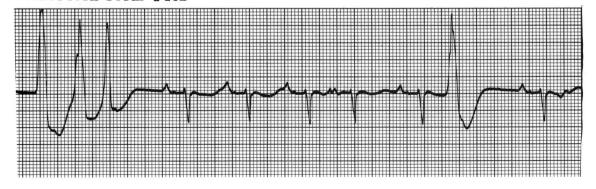

PRACTICE STRIP #103

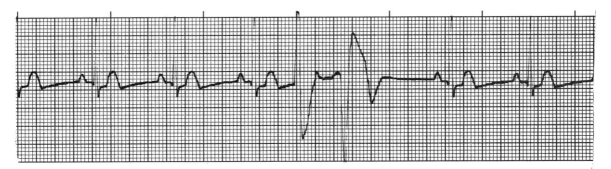

PRACTICE STRIP #104

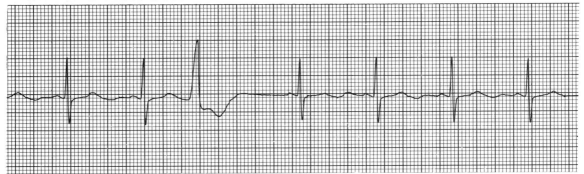

PRACTICE STRIP #105

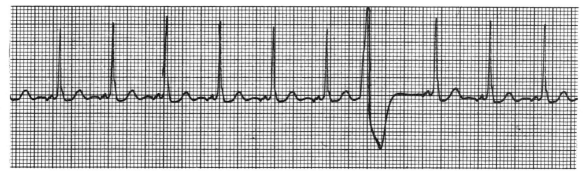

PRACTICE STRIP #106

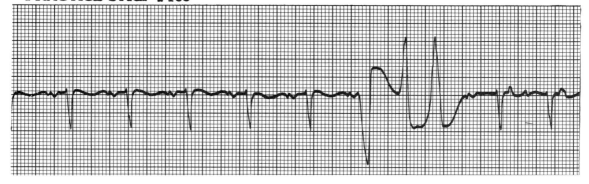

PRACTICE STRIP #107

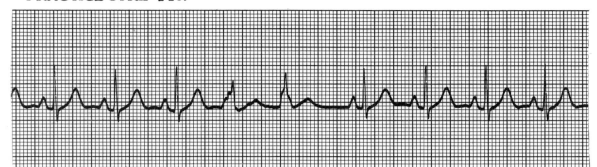

PRACTICE STRIP #108

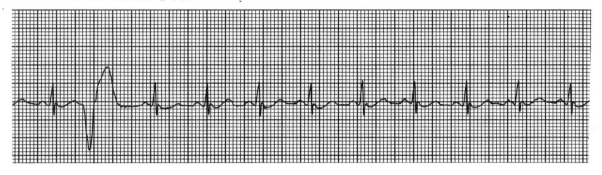

PRACTICE STRIP #109

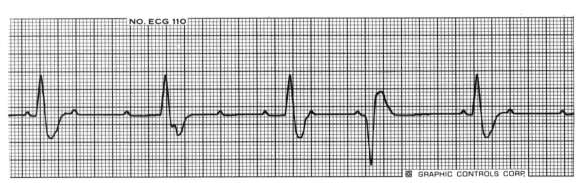

PRACTICE STRIP #110

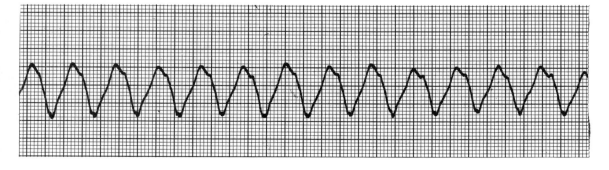

PRACTICE STRIP #111

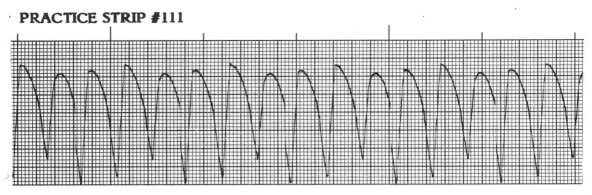

PRACTICE STRIP #112

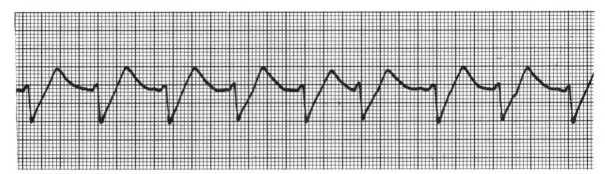

PRACTICE STRIP #113

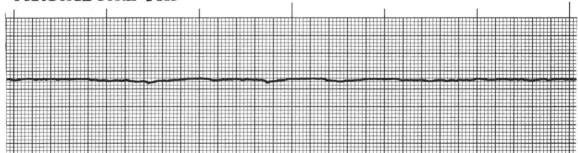

PRACTICE STRIP #114

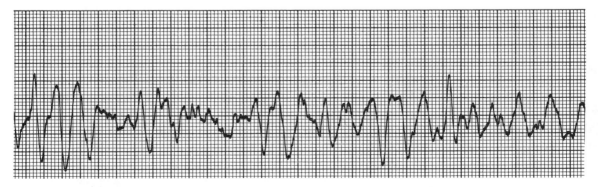

PRACTICE STRIP #115

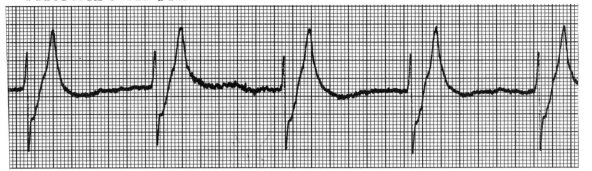

PRACTICE STRIP #116

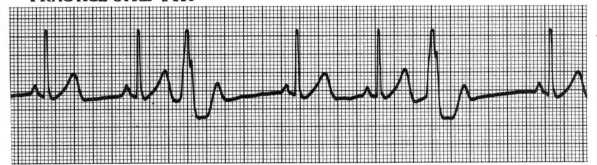

PRACTICE STRIP #117

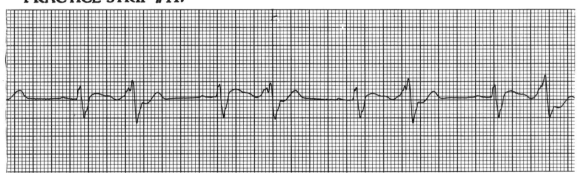
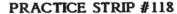

PRACTICE STRIP #118

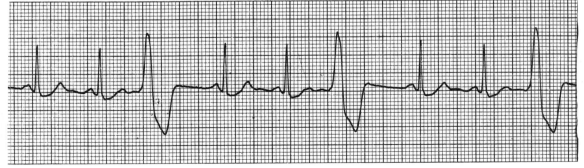

PRACTICE STRIP #119

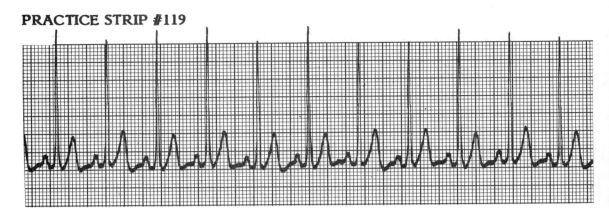

PRACTICE STRIP #120

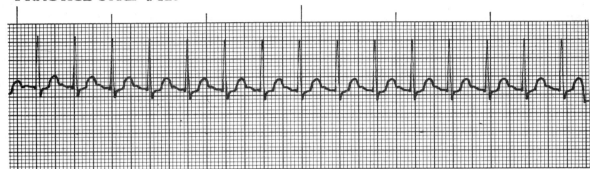

PRACTICE STRIP #121

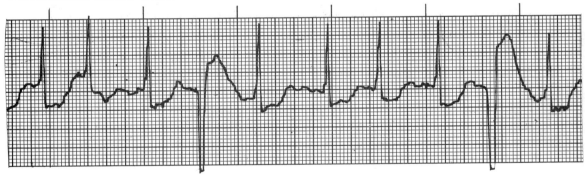

PRACTICE STRIP #122

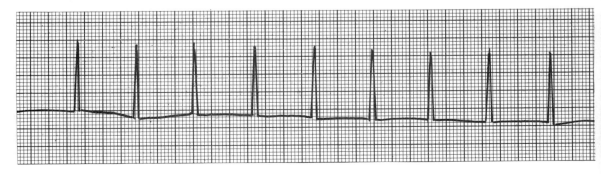

PRACTICE STRIP #123

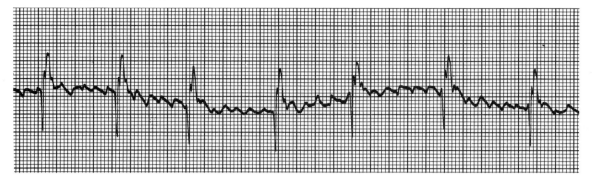

PRACTICE STRIP #124

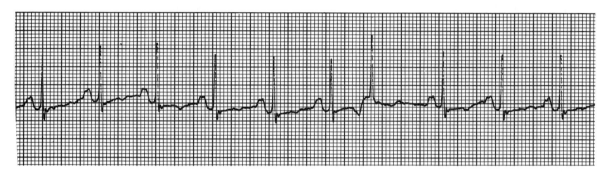

PRACTICE STRIP #125

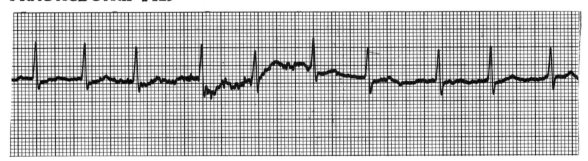

PRACTICE STRIP #126

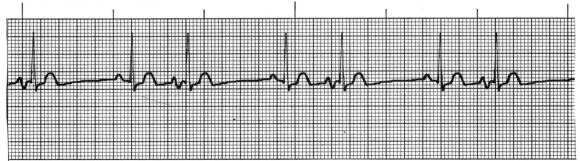

PRACTICE STRIP #127

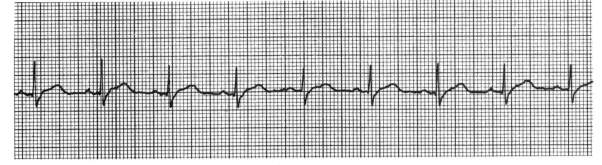

PRACTICE STRIP #128

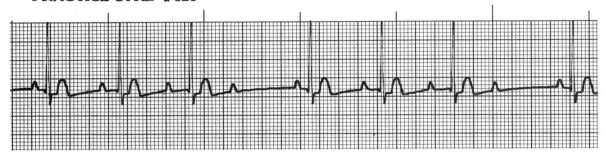

PRACTICE STRIP #129

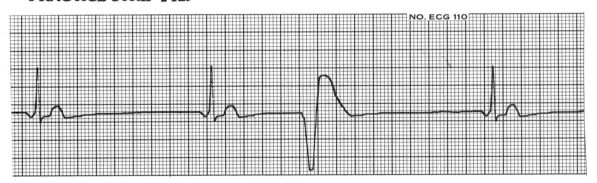

NO. ECG 110

PRACTICE STRIP #130

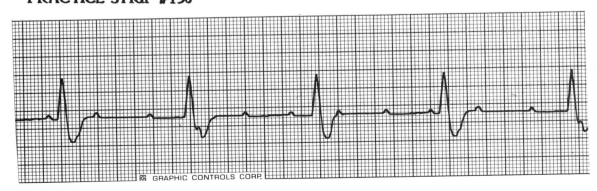

© GRAPHIC CONTROLS CORP.

PRACTICE STRIP #131

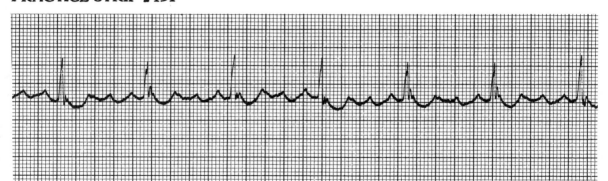

PRACTICE STRIP #132

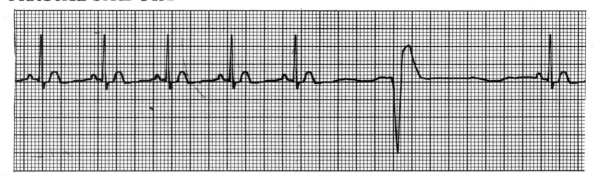

PRACTICE STRIP #133

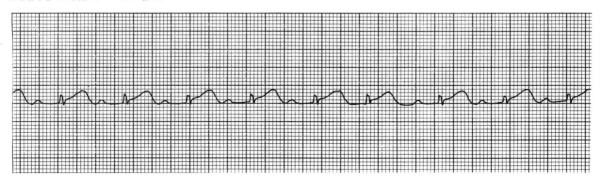

PRACTICE STRIP #134

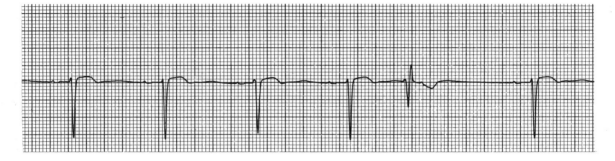

PRACTICE STRIP #135

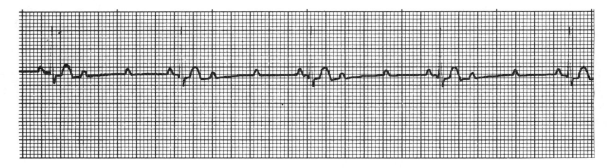

PRACTICE STRIP #136

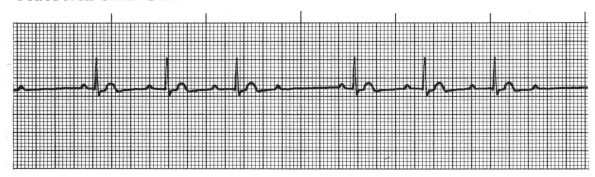

PRACTICE STRIP #137

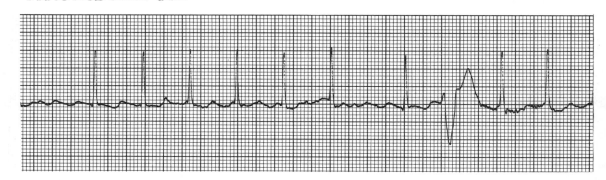

PRACTICE STRIP #138

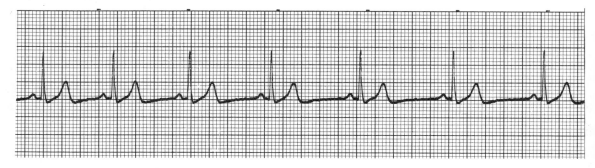

PRACTICE STRIP #139

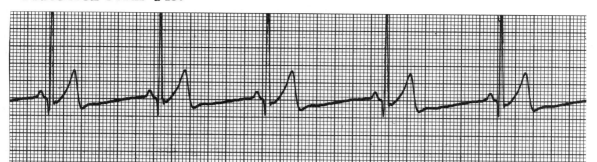

PRACTICE STRIP #140

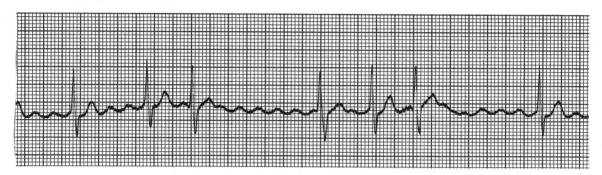

PRACTICE STRIP #141

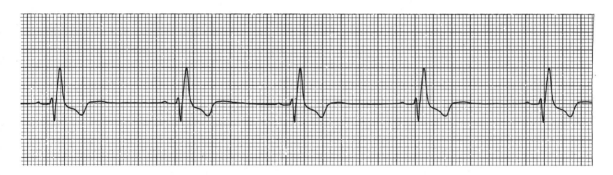

PRACTICE STRIP #142

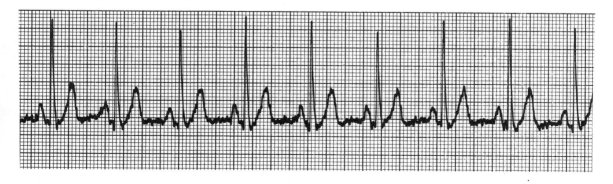

PRACTICE STRIP #143

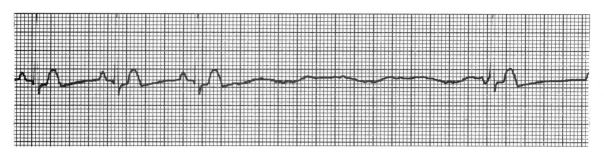

PRACTICE STRIP #144

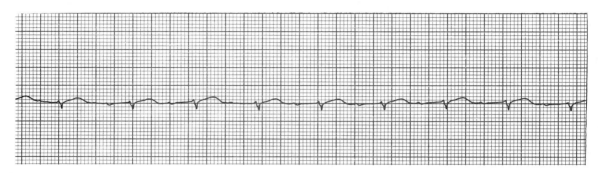

PRACTICE STRIP #145

NO. ECG 110

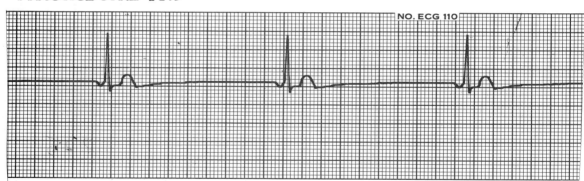

PRACTICE STRIP #146

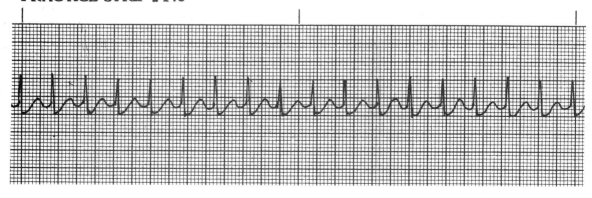

PRACTICE STRIP #147

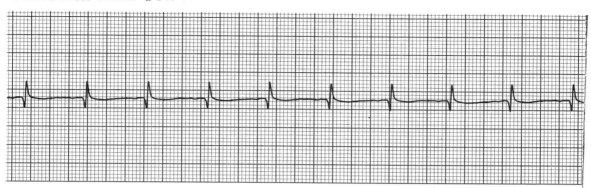

PRACTICE STRIP #148

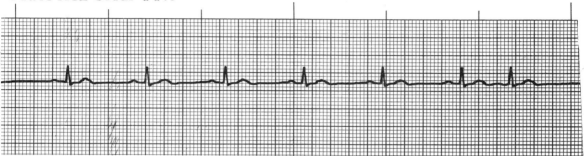

PRACTICE STRIP #149

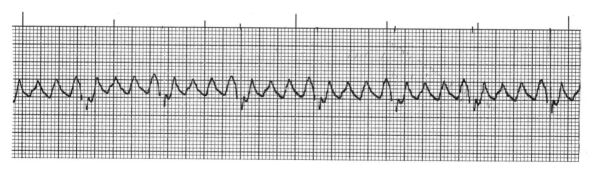

PRACTICE STRIP #150

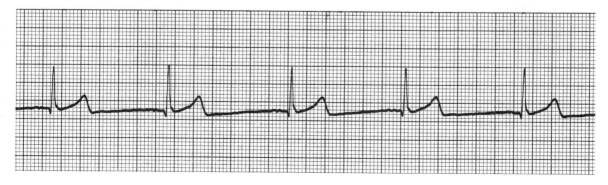

PRACTICE STRIP #151

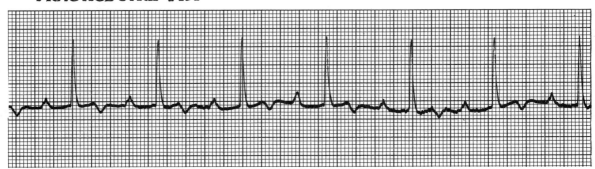

PRACTICE STRIP #152

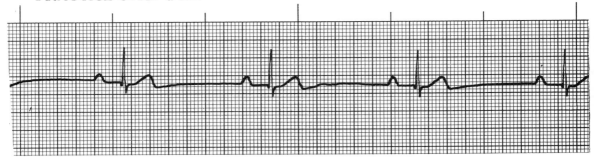

PRACTICE STRIP #153

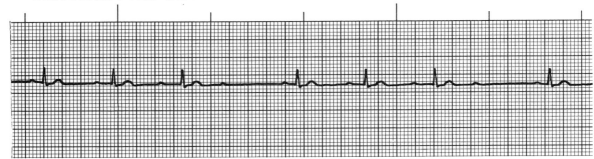

PRACTICE STRIP #154

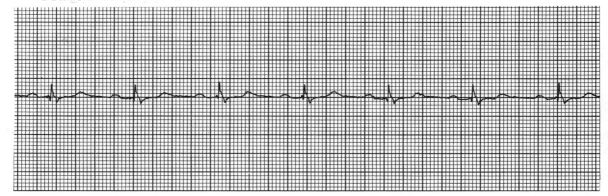

PRACTICE STRIP #155

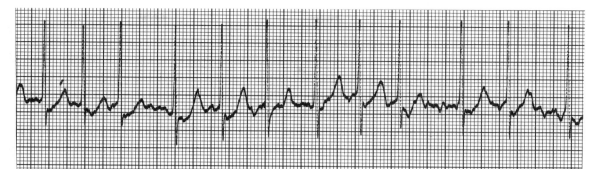

PRACTICE STRIP #156

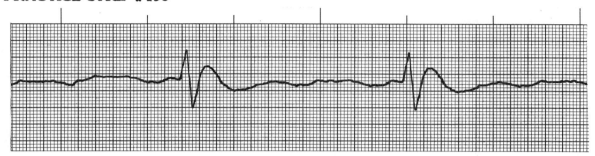

PRACTICE STRIP #157

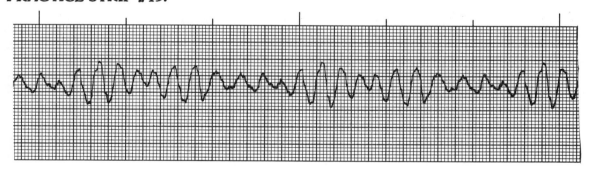

PRACTICE STRIP #158

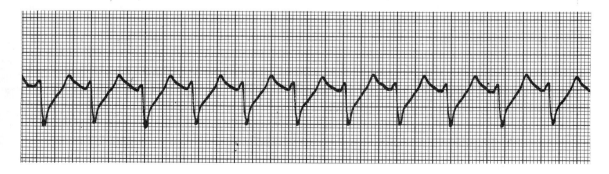

PRACTICE STRIP #159

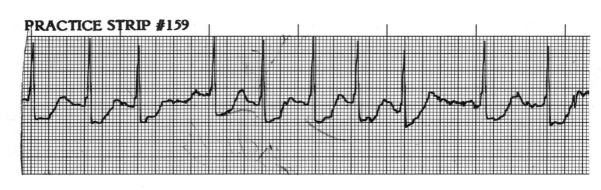

PRACTICE STRIP #160

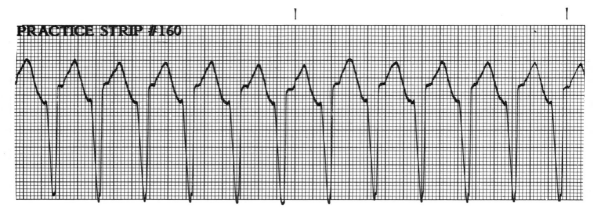

PRACTICE STRIP #161

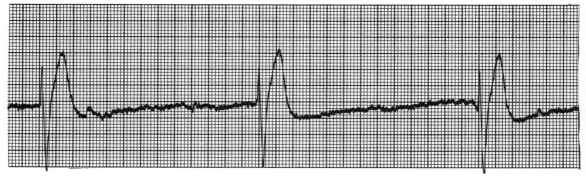

PRACTICE STRIP #162

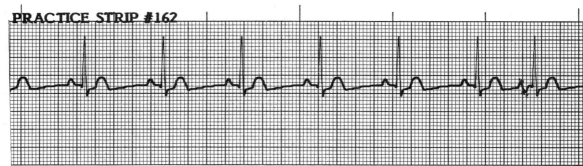

PRACTICE STRIP #163

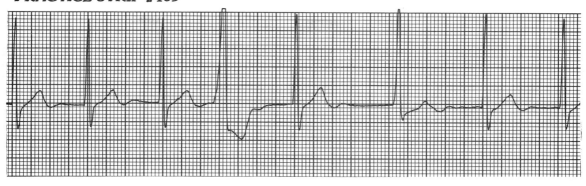

PRACTICE STRIP #164

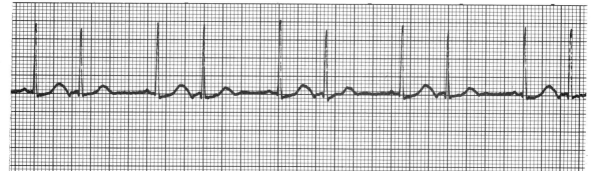

PRACTICE STRIP #165

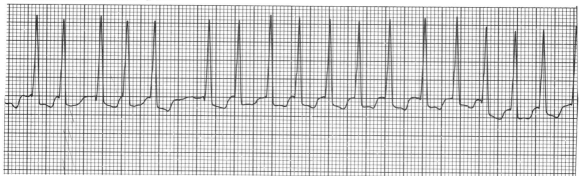

PRACTICE STRIP #166

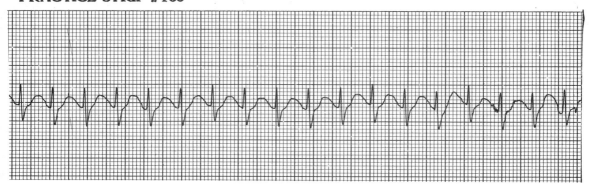

PRACTICE STRIP #167

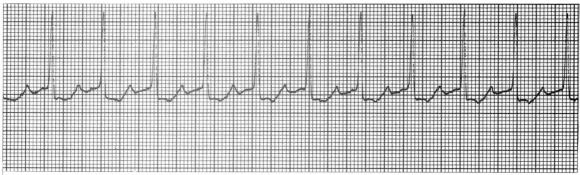

PRACTICE STRIP #168

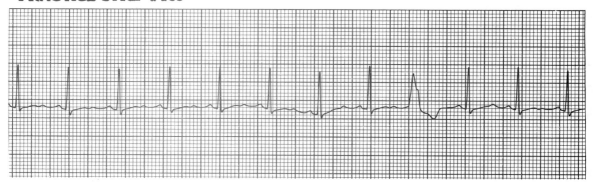

PRACTICE STRIP #169

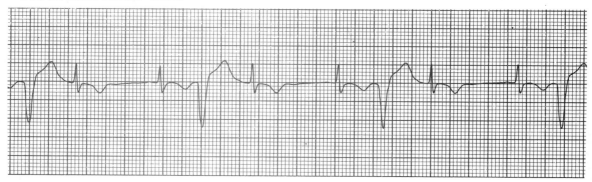

PRACTICE STRIP #170

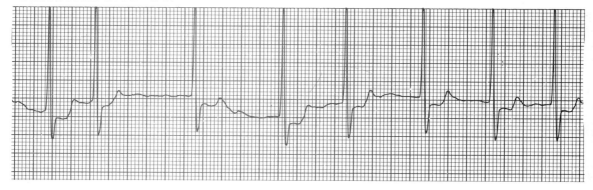

PRACTICE STRIP #171

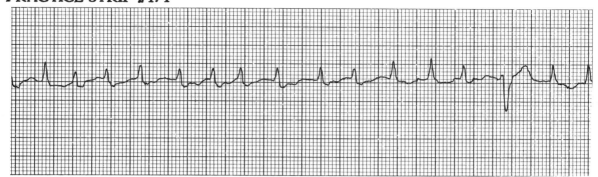

PRACTICE STRIP #172

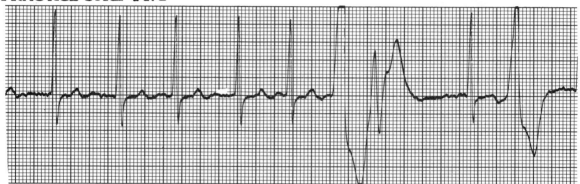

PRACTICE STRIP #173

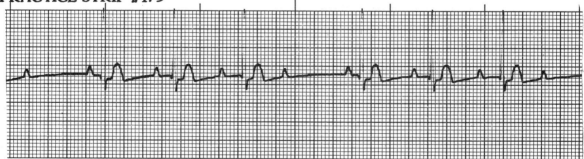

PRACTICE STRIP #174

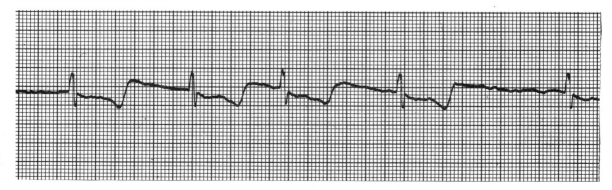

PRACTICE STRIP #175

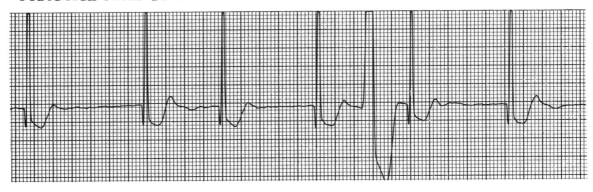

PRACTICE STRIP #176

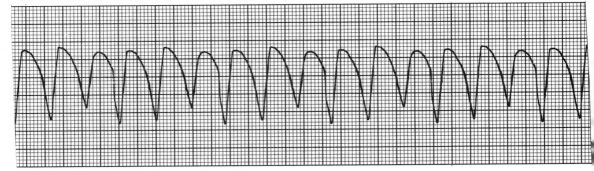

PRACTICE STRIP #177

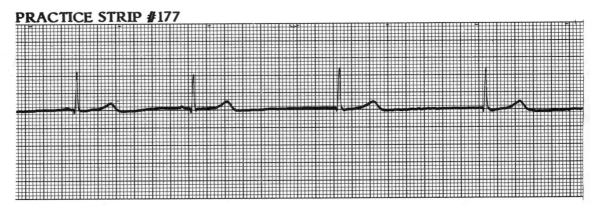

PRACTICE STRIP #178

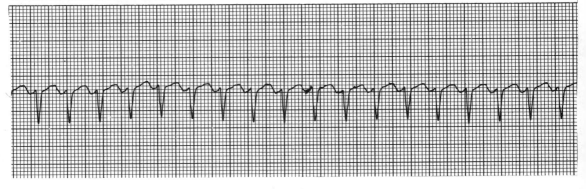

PRACTICE STRIP #179

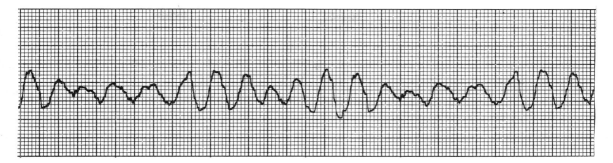

PRACTICE STRIP #180

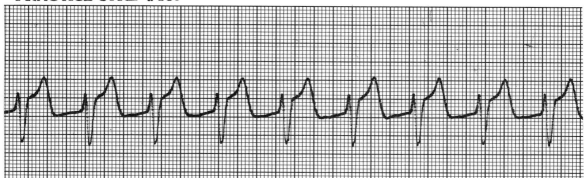

PRACTICE STRIP #181

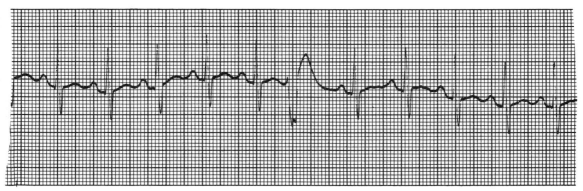

PRACTICE STRIP #182

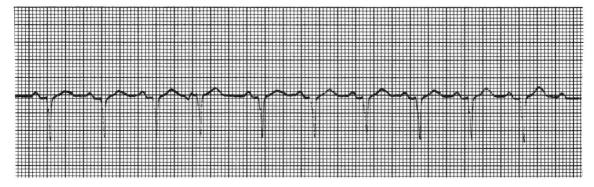

PRACTICE STRIP #183

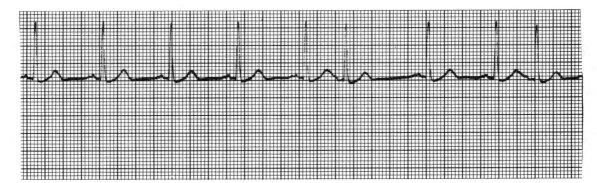

PRACTICE STRIP #184

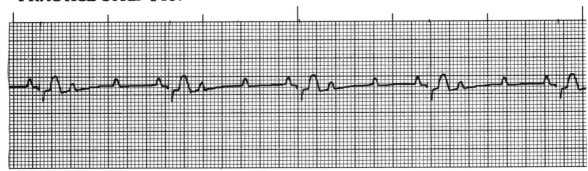

PRACTICE STRIP #185

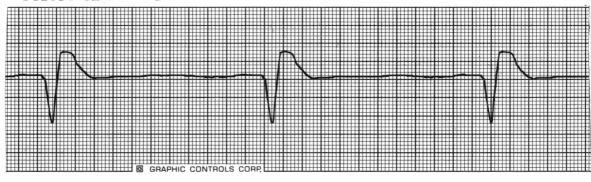

© GRAPHIC CONTROLS CORP.

PRACTICE STRIP #186

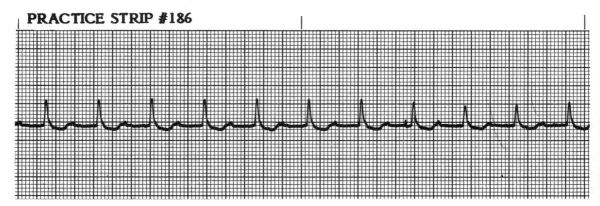

PRACTICE STRIP #187

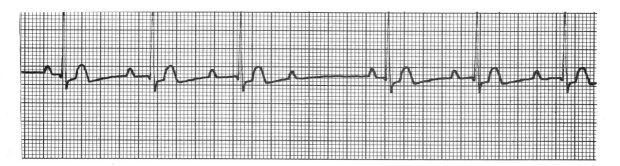

PRACTICE STRIP #188

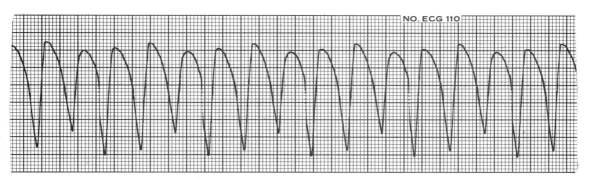

NO. ECG 110

PRACTICE STRIP #189

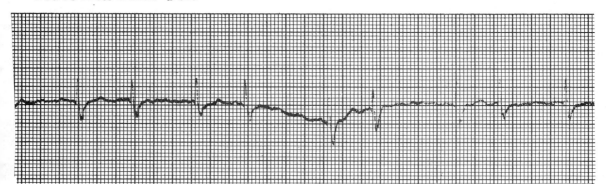

PRACTICE STRIP #190

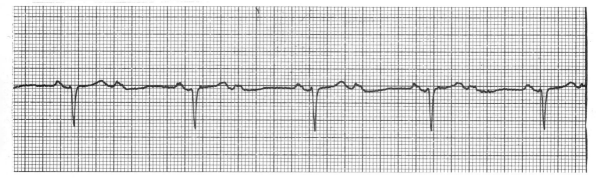

PRACTICE STRIP #191

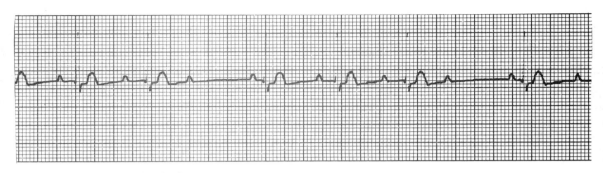

PRACTICE STRIP #192

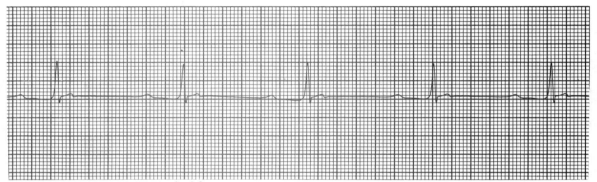

PRACTICE STRIP #193

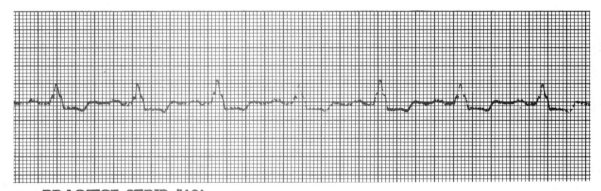

PRACTICE STRIP #194

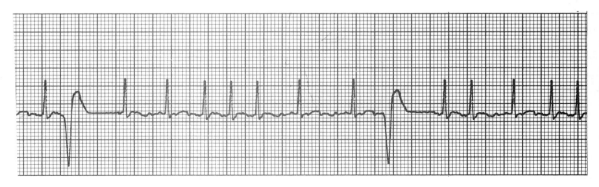

PRACTICE STRIP #195

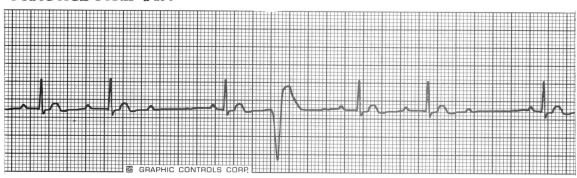

PRACTICE STRIP #196

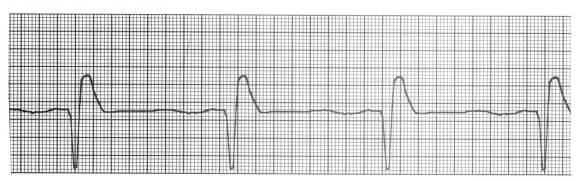

PRACTICE STRIP #197

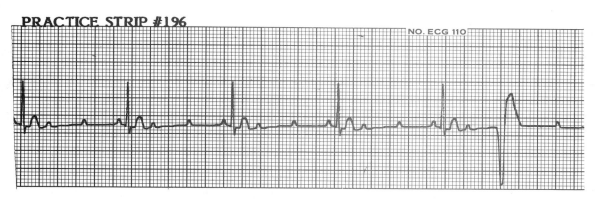

PRACTICE STRIP #198

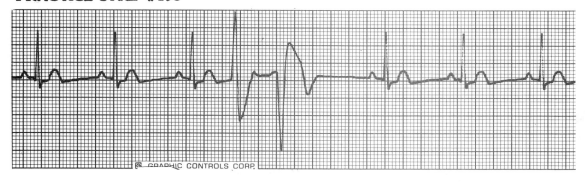

PRACTICE STRIP #199

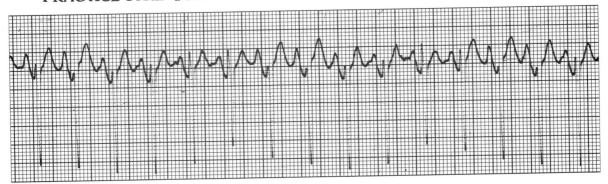

PRACTICE STRIP #200

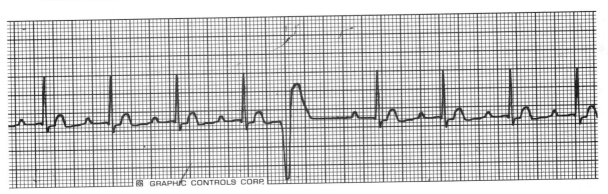

G GRAPHIC CONTROLS CORP.

ANSWERS TO PRACTICE STRIPS

PRACTICE STRIP #97

Atrial Rhythm:	Irregular
Ventricular Rhythm:	Irregular
Atrial Rate:	90 (one P hidden in bizarre complex)
Ventricular Rate:	90
P Waves:	Present and uniform except for the 3rd beat
PRI:	.12 seconds
QRS:	.08 seconds except for the 3rd beat which is greater than .12 seconds
Interpretation:	Sinus Arrhythmia with one PVC

ANSWERS TO PRACTICE STRIPS

PRACTICE STRIP #98

Atrial Rhythm:	Regular except for the 1st and 3rd beats
Ventricular Rhythm:	Regular except for the 1st and 3rd beats
Atrial Rate:	83 (Small Box Method)
Ventricular Rate:	83 (Small Box Method)
P Waves:	Present and inverted before the complex except for the 1st and 3rd beats
PRI:	.08 seconds, constant
QRS:	.08 seconds except for the 1st and 3rd beats which are greater than .12 seconds
Interpretation:	Accelerated Junctional Rhythm with two PVC's (Multifocal)

PRACTICE STRIP #99

Atrial Rhythm:	Unable to identify P wave
Ventricular Rhythm:	Irregular
Atrial Rate:	0
Ventricular Rate:	100
P Waves:	0
PRI:	0
QRS:	.10 seconds except for the 4th and 8th beats which are greater than .12 seconds
Interpretation:	Atrial Fibrillation with two PVC's

PRACTICE STRIP #100

Atrial Rhythm:	Irregular
Ventricular Rhythm:	Irregular
Atrial Rate:	50
Ventricular Rate:	60
P Waves:	Present and uniform except for the 2nd beat where it is absent
PRI:	.12 seconds, constant
QRS:	.08 seconds except for the 2nd beat which is .16 seconds
Interpretation:	Sinus Arrhythmia with one Ventricular Escape Beat (Remember premature beats occur early in the cycle; escape beats occur late. The second beat in this strip is not early--it is late; therefore, it is an escape beat.)

-219-

ANSWERS TO PRACTICE STRIPS

PRACTICE STRIP #101

Atrial Rhythm:	Irregular
Ventricular Rhythm:	Irregular
Atrial Rate:	50
Ventricular Rate:	70
P Waves:	Present except for the 4th and 7th beats where it is lost in the complex
PRI:	.14 seconds, constant
QRS:	.08 seconds except for the 4th and 7th beats which are greater than .12 seconds
Interpretation:	Sinus Arrhythmia with two PVC's

PRACTICE STRIP #102

Atrial Rhythm:	Irregular
Ventricular Rhythm:	Irregular
Atrial Rate:	100
Ventricular Rate:	100
P Waves:	Some are hidden in the large ventricular complexes (1st, 2nd, 3rd & 9th P waves are hidden). The 7th beat has a P that looks very different from the other P's and it is early.
PRI:	.26 seconds when present
QRS:	.10 seconds except for the 1st, 2nd, 3rd and 9th beats which are greater than .12 seconds
Interpretation:	Run of Ventricular Tachycardia, RSR with First Degree A-V Heart Block, one PAC (7th beat) and one PVC (9th beat)

PRACTICE STRIP #103

Atrial Rhythm:	Regular except for the 4th and 5th beats
Ventricular Rhythm:	Regular except for the 4th and 5th beats
Atrial Rate:	75 (Small Box Method)
Ventricular Rate:	75 (Small Box Method)
P Waves:	Present except for the 4th and 5th beats
PRI:	.16 seconds, constant
QRS:	.10 seconds except for the 4th and 5th beats which are greater than .12 seconds
Interpretation:	RSR with two Multifocal PVC's

ANSWERS TO PRACTICE STRIPS

PRACTICE STRIP #104

Atrial Rhythm:	Regular except for the 3rd beat
Ventricular Rhythm:	Regular except for the 3rd beat
Atrial Rate:	70
Ventricular Rate:	70
P Waves:	Present, one P/complex, except for the 3rd beat
PRI:	.12 seconds
QRS:	.08 seconds except for the 3rd beat which is greater than .12 seconds
Interpretation:	RSR with one PVC

PRACTICE STRIP #105

Atrial Rhythm:	Regular except for the 7th beat
Ventricular Rhythm:	Regular except for the 7th beat
Atrial Rate:	100
Ventricular Rate:	100
P Waves:	Present and uniform except for the 7th beat where it is absent (notice the biphasic contour of the P wave; it is negative then positive)
PRI:	.12 seconds, constant
QRS:	.08 seconds except for the 7th beat which is greater than .12 seconds
Interpretation:	RSR with one PVC

PRACTICE STRIP #106

Atrial Rhythm:	Regular except for the run starting with the 6th beat
Ventricular Rhythm:	Regular except for the run starting with the 6th beat
Atrial Rate:	94 (Small Box Method)
Ventricular Rate:	100 (Small Box Method)
P Waves:	Present with notched appearance
PRI:	.24 seconds, constant
QRS:	.10 seconds except for the 7th, 8th and 9th beats where it is greater than .12 seconds
Interpretation:	RSR with First Degree A-V Heart Block and Run of Multifocal Ventricular Tachycardia

ANSWERS TO PRACTICE STRIPS

PRACTICE STRIP #107

Atrial Rhythm:	Regular except for the 4th and 5th beats
Ventricular Rhythm:	Regular except for the 4th and 5th beats
Atrial Rate:	94 (Small Box Method)
Ventricular Rate:	90 (Six-Second Method)
P Waves:	Present and uniform, one P/complex, except for the 4th and 5th beats
PRI:	.16 seconds, constant
QRS:	.08 seconds except for the 4th and 5th beats which are greater than .12 seconds
Interpretation:	RSR with Sequential and Multifocal PVC's

PRACTICE STRIP #108

Atrial Rhythm:	Regular except for the 2nd beat
Ventricular Rhythm:	Regular except for the 2nd beat
Atrial Rate:	107 (Small Box Method)
Ventricular Rate:	110
P Waves:	Present, one P/complex except for the 2nd beat
PRI:	.12 seconds, constant
QRS:	.06 seconds except for the 2nd beat which is greater than .12 seconds
Interpretation:	Sinus Tachycardia with one PVC

PRACTICE STRIP #109

Atrial Rhythm:	Regular
Ventricular Rhythm:	Regular
Atrial Rate:	110
Ventricular Rate:	50
P Waves:	Present, more P's than complexes
PRI:	Variable
QRS:	All greater than .12 seconds, 4th complex looks different than the others and it is early
Interpretation:	CHB with PVC

ANSWERS TO PRACTICE STRIPS
PRACTICE STRIP #110

Atrial Rhythm:	Ø
Ventricular Rhythm:	Regular
Atrial Rate:	Ø
Ventricular Rate:	130
P Waves:	Ø
PRI:	Ø
QRS:	Extremely wide and bizarre
Interpretation:	Ventricular Tachycardia

PRACTICE STRIP #111

Atrial Rhythm:	Ø
Ventricular Rhythm:	Regular
Atrial Rate:	Ø
Ventricular Rate:	160
P Waves:	Ø
PRI:	Ø
QRS:	Greater than .12 seconds
Interpretation:	Ventricular Tachycardia

PRACTICE STRIP #112

Atrial Rhythm:	Ø
Ventricular Rhythm:	Slightly irregular
Atrial Rate:	Ø
Ventricular Rate:	90
P Waves:	Ø
PRI:	Ø
QRS:	.24 seconds
Interpretation:	Accelerated Ventricular Rhythm

ANSWERS TO PRACTICE STRIPS
PRACTICE STRIP #113

Atrial Rhythm:	∅
Ventricular Rhythm:	∅
Atrial Rate:	∅
Ventricular Rate:	∅
P Waves:	∅
PRI:	∅
QRS:	∅
Interpretation:	Asystole

PRACTICE STRIP #114

Atrial Rhythm:	Totally chaotic rhythm
Ventricular Rhythm:	Totally chaotic rhythm
Atrial Rate:	∅
Ventricular Rate:	∅
P Waves:	∅
PRI:	∅
QRS:	∅
Interpretation:	Ventricular Fibrillation

PRACTICE STRIP #115

Atrial Rhythm:	∅
Ventricular Rhythm:	Regular
Atrial Rate:	∅
Ventricular Rate:	43
P Waves:	∅
PRI:	∅
QRS:	Greater than .12 seconds
Interpretation:	Idioventricular Rhythm

PRACTICE STRIP #116

Atrial Rhythm:	Every 3rd beat is a PVC
Ventricular Rhythm:	Every 3rd beat is a PVC
Atrial Rate:	70 (some P's are lost in the PVC's)
Ventricular Rate:	70
P Waves:	Present except every 3rd beat
PRI:	.16 seconds
QRS:	.06 seconds except for every 3rd beat which are greater than .12 seconds
Interpretation:	Ventricular Trigeminy

PRACTICE STRIP #117

Atrial Rhythm:	Every other beat is premature
Ventricular Rhythm:	Irregular
Atrial Rate:	80
Ventricular Rate:	80 (Six-Second Strip)
P Waves:	Every other one is hidden in the premature beat
PRI:	.20 seconds
QRS:	.10 seconds/.22 seconds
Interpretation:	Ventricular Bigeminy

PRACTICE STRIP #118

Atrial Rhythm:	Regular except for every 3rd beat
Ventricular Rhythm:	Regular except for every 3rd beat
Atrial Rate:	90
Ventricular Rate:	90
P Waves:	Present except for every 3rd beat
PRI:	.12 seconds, constant when present
QRS:	.06 seconds except for every 3rd beat which are greater than .12 seconds
Interpretation:	Ventricular Trigeminy

ANSWERS TO PRACTICE STRIPS

PRACTICE STRIP #119

Atrial Rhythm:	Regular
Ventricular Rhythm:	Regular
Atrial Rate:	110
Ventricular Rate:	110
P Waves:	Present, one P/complex, uniform
PRI:	.14 seconds, constant
QRS:	.08 seconds
Interpretation:	Sinus Tachycardia

PRACTICE STRIP #120

Atrial Rhythm:	Regular
Ventricular Rhythm:	Regular
Atrial Rate:	150
Ventricular Rate:	150
P Waves:	Present, one P/complex
PRI:	.16 seconds
QRS:	.08 seconds
Interpretation:	Sinus Tachycardia

PRACTICE STRIP #121

Atrial Rhythm:	Unable to identify P wave
Ventricular Rhythm:	Irregular
Atrial Rate:	0
Ventricular Rate:	100
P Waves:	0
PRI:	0
QRS:	.08 seconds except for the 4th and 9th beats which are wide and bizarre
Interpretation:	Atrial Fibrillation, Controlled and two PVC's

ANSWERS TO PRACTICE STRIPS

PRACTICE STRIP #122

Atrial Rhythm:	Ø
Ventricular Rhythm:	Regular
Atrial Rate:	Ø
Ventricular Rate:	90
P Waves:	Ø
PRI:	Ø
QRS:	.06 seconds
Interpretation:	Accelerated Junctional Rhythm

PRACTICE STRIP #123

Atrial Rhythm:	Regular
Ventricular Rhythm:	Irregular
Atrial Rate:	375
Ventricular Rate:	70
P Waves:	Flutter waves are present
PRI:	Ø
QRS:	.12 seconds
Interpretation:	Atrial Flutter with Variable and Aberrant Conduction

PRACTICE STRIP #124

Atrial Rhythm:	Regular except for the 7th beat
Ventricular Rhythm:	Regular except for the 7th beat
Atrial Rate:	100
Ventricular Rate:	100
P Waves:	Present and uniform except for the 7th beat
PRI:	.16 seconds, constant
QRS:	.06 seconds
Interpretation:	RSR with one PAC

ANSWERS TO PRACTICE STRIPS

PRACTICE STRIP #125

Atrial Rhythm:	Unable to identify P wave
Ventricular Rhythm:	Irregular
Atrial Rate:	$\emptyset$
Ventricular Rate:	100
P Waves:	$\emptyset$
PRI:	$\emptyset$
QRS:	.08 seconds
Interpretation:	Atrial Fibrillation, Controlled

PRACTICE STRIP #126

Atrial Rhythm:	Irregular, every other beat is early
Ventricular Rhythm:	Irregular, every other beat is early
Atrial Rate:	70
Ventricular Rate:	70
P Waves:	Present, one P/complex, early P's are different than sinus P
PRI:	.16 seconds, constant
QRS:	.08 seconds
Interpretation:	Atrial Bigeminy

PRACTICE STRIP #127

Atrial Rhythm:	Regular
Ventricular Rhythm:	Regular
Atrial Rate:	90
Ventricular Rate:	90
P Waves:	Present, one P/complex with different configurations
PRI:	.18 seconds, constant
QRS:	.08 seconds
Interpretation:	Wandering Pacemaker

ANSWERS TO PRACTICE STRIPS
PRACTICE STRIP #128

Atrial Rhythm:	Regular
Ventricular Rhythm:	Irregular
Atrial Rate:	90
Ventricular Rate:	70
P Waves:	Present, more P's than complexes
PRI:	.14 seconds to .24 seconds, variable with a pattern
QRS:	.08 seconds
Interpretation:	Mobitz I

PRACTICE STRIP #129

Atrial Rhythm:	Ø
Ventricular Rhythm:	Regular
Atrial Rate:	32 (Small Box Method)
Ventricular Rate:	40
P Waves:	Present and inverted before the complex
PRI:	.08 seconds
QRS:	.10 seconds
Interpretation:	Junctional Bradycardia with one PVC

PRACTICE STRIP #130

Atrial Rhythm:	Regular
Ventricular Rhythm:	Regular
Atrial Rate:	110 (Count the one lost in the ST segment)
Ventricular Rate:	50
P Waves:	Present, more P's than complexes
PRI:	Variable
QRS:	Greater than .12 seconds
Interpretation:	CHB

ANSWERS TO PRACTICE STRIPS

PRACTICE STRIP #131

Atrial Rhythm:	Regular
Ventricular Rhythm:	Regular
Atrial Rate:	270
Ventricular Rate:	70
P Waves:	Flutter waves
PRI:	0
QRS:	.08 seconds
Interpretation:	Atrial Flutter 4:1

PRACTICE STRIP #132

Atrial Rhythm:	Regular until the pause
Ventricular Rhythm:	Regular until the pause
Atrial Rate:	60
Ventricular Rate:	70
P Waves:	Present and uniform except for the 6th beat
PRI:	.12 seconds
QRS:	.08 seconds except for the 6th beat which is greater than .12 seconds
Interpretation:	RSR with Sinus Arrest and Ventricular Escape Beat. Sinus node regains control.

PRACTICE STRIP #133

Atrial Rhythm:	Regular except for 6th beat
Ventricular Rhythm:	Regular except for 6th beat
Atrial Rate:	90
Ventricular Rate:	90
P Waves:	Present and uniform except for 6th beat where it is absent
PRI:	.28 seconds, constant
QRS:	.06 seconds
Interpretation:	RSR with First Degree A-V Heart Block and one PJC (Notice the elevated ST segment)

PRACTICE STRIP #134

Atrial Rhythm:	Regular except for the 5th beat
Ventricular Rhythm:	Regular except for the 5th beat
Atrial Rate:	60
Ventricular Rate:	60
P Waves:	Present and uniform
PRI:	.20 seconds, constant
QRS:	.06 seconds except for the 5th complex
Interpretation:	RSR with one PVC (This is a good illustration of why the sinus rhythm remains regular during PVC's. This particular PVC is small enough that it lets us see what happens to the sinus with PVC's. March the P waves out with your calipers and you will see the 5th one is right on time after the PVC. The rhythm of the sinus node is not interrupted by the PVC and this is what causes the compensatory pause.)

PRACTICE STRIP #135

Atrial Rhythm:	Regular
Ventricular Rhythm:	Regular
Atrial Rate:	130
Ventricular Rate:	50
P Waves:	Present, more P's than complexes
PRI:	.12 seconds, constant
QRS:	.08 seconds
Interpretation:	Mobitz II

PRACTICE STRIP #136

Atrial Rhythm:	Regular
Ventricular Rhythm:	Irregular
Atrial Rate:	90
Ventricular Rate:	60
P Waves:	Present, more P's than complexes
PRI:	Variable with a pattern of progressively longer until one P does not conduct to the ventricles
QRS:	.08 seconds
Interpretation:	Mobitz I

PRACTICE STRIP #137

Atrial Rhythm:	Unable to identify P wave
Ventricular Rhythm:	Irregular
Atrial Rate:	0
Ventricular Rate:	100
P Waves:	0
PRI:	0
QRS:	.06 seconds except for the 8th beat which is greater than .12 seconds
Interpretation:	Atrial Fibrillatiion, Controlled, with one PVC

PRACTICE STRIP #138

Atrial Rhythm:	Irregular
Ventricular Rhythm:	Irregular
Atrial Rate:	70
Ventricular Rate:	70
P Waves:	Present, one P/complex, uniform
PRI:	.12 seconds,
QRS:	.08 seconds
Interpretation:	Sinus Arrhythmia

PRACTICE STRIP #139

Atrial Rhythm:	Regular
Ventricular Rhythm:	Regular
Atrial Rate:	50
Ventricular Rate:	50
P Waves:	Present, one P/complex, uniform
PRI:	.12 seconds, constant
QRS:	.08 seconds
Interpretation:	Sinus Bradycardia

ANSWERS TO PRACTICE STRIPS
PRACTICE STRIP #140

Atrial Rhythm:	Regular
Ventricular Rhythm:	Irregular
Atrial Rate:	300
Ventricular Rate:	70
P Waves:	Flutter waves are present
PRI:	Ø
QRS:	.11 seconds
Interpretation:	Atrial Flutter with Variable Conduction

PRACTICE STRIP #141

Atrial Rhythm:	Regular
Ventricular Rhythm:	Regular
Atrial Rate:	50
Ventricular Rate:	50
P Waves:	Present, one P/complex, uniform
PRI:	.14 seconds, constant
QRS:	.12 seconds
Interpretation:	Sinus Bradycardia with Aberrant Ventricular Conduction

PRACTICE STRIP #142

Atrial Rhythm:	Regular
Ventricular Rhythm:	Regular
Atrial Rate:	90
Ventricular Rate:	90
P Waves:	Present, one P/complex, uniform
PRI:	.16 seconds, constant
QRS:	.10 seconds
Interpretation:	RSR

ANSWERS TO PRACTICE STRIPS

PRACTICE STRIP #143

Atrial Rhythm:	Regular, until the arrest
Ventricular Rhythm:	Regular, until the arrest
Atrial Rate:	65 (Small Box Method)
Ventricular Rate:	40 (Six Second Method)
P Waves:	Present until the arrest, inverted before the 4th complex
PRI:	.16 seconds, constant except the 4th beat where PRI is .0? seconds
QRS:	.08 seconds
Interpretation:	RSR with Sinus Arrest and Junctional Escape Beat

PRACTICE STRIP #144

Atrial Rhythm:	Regular
Ventricular Rhythm:	Regular
Atrial Rate:	90
Ventricular Rate:	90
P Waves:	Present (very small in this lead)
PRI:	.24 seconds, constant
QRS:	.08 seconds (very small; this is not a very good lead to see what is going on with this patient)
Interpretation:	RSR with First Degree A-V Heart Block

PRACTICE STRIP #145

Atrial Rhythm:	Regular
Ventricular Rhythm:	Regular
Atrial Rate:	30
Ventricular Rate:	30
P Waves:	Present and uniform, inverted before the complex
PRI:	.08 seconds, constant
QRS:	.08 seconds
Interpretation:	Junctional Bradycardia

ANSWERS TO PRACTICE STRIPS

PRACTICE STRIP #146

Atrial Rhythm:	Regular
Ventricular Rhythm:	Regular
Atrial Rate:	170
Ventricular Rate:	170
P Waves:	Unable to ascertain if those are T's or P's on T's
PRI:	Normal if they are present
QRS:	.08 seconds
Interpretation:	Supraventricular Tachycardia (SVT)

PRACTICE STRIP #147

Atrial Rhythm:	∅
Ventricular Rhythm:	Regular
Atrial Rate:	∅
Ventricular Rate:	100
P Waves:	∅
PRI:	∅
QRS:	.10 seconds
Interpretation:	Accelerated Junctional Rhythm

PRACTICE STRIP #148

Atrial Rhythm:	Regular except for the 7th beat
Ventricular Rhythm:	Regular except for the 7th beat
Atrial Rate:	70
Ventricular Rate:	70
P Waves:	Present and uniform except for the 7th one which is absent
PRI:	.16 seconds, constant
QRS:	.06 seconds
Interpretation:	RSR with one PJC

PRACTICE STRIP #149

Atrial Rhythm:	Regular
Ventricular Rhythm:	Regular
Atrial Rate:	300
Ventricular Rate:	70
P Waves:	Flutter waves are present
PRI:	Ø
QRS:	.08 seconds
Interpretation:	Atrial Flutter 4:1

PRACTICE STRIP #150

Atrial Rhythm:	Regular
Ventricular Rhythm:	Regular
Atrial Rate:	Ø
Ventricular Rate:	50
P Waves:	Very small, inverted before the complex
PRI:	.12 seconds
QRS:	.08 seconds
Interpretation:	Junctional Escape Rhythm (If you did not see those tiny inverted P waves, you still should have been able to make the interpretation.)

PRACTICE STRIP #151

Atrial Rhythm:	Regular
Ventricular Rhythm:	Regular
Atrial Rate:	70
Ventricular Rate:	70
P Waves:	Present, one P/complex, uniform
PRI:	.32 seconds, constant
QRS:	.08 seconds
Interpretation:	RSR with First Degree A-V Heart Block

ANSWERS TO PRACTICE STRIPS

PRACTICE STRIP #152

Atrial Rhythm:	Regular
Ventricular Rhythm:	Regular
Atrial Rate:	40
Ventricular Rate:	40
P Waves:	Present, one P/complex, uniform
PRI:	.28 seconds, constant
QRS:	.08 seconds
Interpretation:	Sinus Bradycardia with First Degree A-V Heart Block

PRACTICE STRIP #153

Atrial Rhythm:	Regular
Ventricular Rhythm:	Irregular
Atrial Rate:	90
Ventricular Rate:	70
P Waves:	Present, more P's than complexes
PRI:	Variable with a pattern; becomes progressively longer until one P does not conduct to the ventricles
QRS:	.04 seconds
Interpretation:	Mobitz I

PRACTICE STRIP #154

Atrial Rhythm:	Regular
Ventricular Rhythm:	Regular
Atrial Rate:	70
Ventricular Rate:	70
P Waves:	Present, one P/complex, uniform
PRI:	.22 seconds, constant
QRS:	.10 seconds
Interpretation:	RSR with First Degree AV Heart Block

ANSWERS TO PRACTICE STRIPS

PRACTICE STRIP #155

Atrial Rhythm:	Unable to identify P wave
Ventricular Rhythm:	Irregular
Atrial Rate:	0
Ventricular Rate:	120
P Waves:	0
PRI:	0
QRS:	.08 seconds
Interpretation:	Atrial Fibrillation, Uncontrolled

PRACTICE STRIP #156

Atrial Rhythm:	0
Ventricular Rhythm:	Unable to tell with just two beats
Atrial Rate:	0
Ventricular Rate:	20
P Waves:	0
PRI:	0
QRS:	.22 seconds
Interpretation:	Idioventricular Rhythm

PRACTICE STRIP #157

Atrial Rhythm:	Totally chaotic rhythm
Ventricular Rhythm:	Totally chaotic rhythm
Atrial Rate:	0
Ventricular Rate:	0
P Waves:	0
PRI:	0
QRS:	0
Interpretation:	Ventricular Fibrillation

ANSWERS TO PRACTICE STRIPS
PRACTICE STRIP #158

Atrial Rhythm:	Ø
Ventricular Rhythm:	Regular
Atrial Rate:	Ø
Ventricular Rate:	110
P Waves:	Ø
PRI:	Ø
QRS:	Very wide and bizarre, greater than .12 seconds
Interpretation:	Ventricular Tachycardia

PRACTICE STRIP #159

Atrial Rhythm:	Unable to identify P wave
Ventricular Rhythm:	Irregular
Atrial Rate:	Ø
Ventricular Rate:	100
P Waves:	Ø
PRI:	Ø
QRS:	.08 seconds
Interpretation:	Atrial Fibrillation, Controlled

PRACTICE STRIP #160

Atrial Rhythm:	Ø
Ventricular Rhythm:	Regular
Atrial Rate:	Ø
Ventricular Rate:	120
P Waves:	Ø
PRI:	Ø
QRS:	Greater than .12 seconds
Interpretation:	Ventricular Tachycardia

ANSWERS TO PRACTICE STRIPS
PRACTICE STRIP #161

Atrial Rhythm:	Ø
Ventricular Rhythm:	Regular
Atrial Rate:	Ø
Ventricular Rate:	30
P Waves:	Absent
PRI:	Ø
QRS:	Greater than .12 seconds
Interpretation:	Idioventricular Rhythm

PRACTICE STRIP #162

Atrial Rhythm:	Regular except for the 7th beat
Ventricular Rhythm:	Regular except for the 7th beat
Atrial Rate:	70
Ventricular Rate:	70
P Waves:	Present, one P/complex, uniform except for the 7th beat which is also early
PRI:	.14 seconds, constant
QRS:	.08 seconds
Interpretation:	RSR with one PAC

PRACTICE STRIP #163

Atrial Rhythm:	Unable to identify P wave
Ventricular Rhythm:	Irregular
Atrial Rate:	Ø
Ventricular Rate:	80
P Waves:	Ø
PRI:	Ø
QRS:	.10 seconds except for the 4th beat which is greater than .12 seconds
Interpretation:	Atrial Fibrillation, Controlled, with one PVC

ANSWERS TO PRACTICE STRIPS

PRACTICE STRIP #164

Atrial Rhythm:	Irregular, every other beat is early
Ventricular Rhythm:	Irregular, every other beat is early
Atrial Rate:	100
Ventricular Rate:	100
P Waves:	Present, every other P is inverted before the complex
PRI:	.10 to .12 seconds
QRS:	.08 seconds
Interpretation:	Junctional Bigeminy

PRACTICE STRIP #165

Atrial Rhythm:	Unable to identify P wave
Ventricular Rhythm:	Irregular
Atrial Rate:	Ø
Ventricular Rate:	170
P Waves:	Ø
PRI:	Ø
QRS:	.10 seconds
Interpretation:	Atrial Fibrillation, Uncontrolled

PRACTICE STRIP #166

Atrial Rhythm:	Regular
Ventricular Rhythm:	Regular
Atrial Rate:	Unable to ascertain
Ventricular Rate:	180
P Waves:	Unable to ascertain if they are present or not
PRI:	Unable to measure
QRS:	.08 seconds
Interpretation:	Supraventricular Tachycardia (SVT)

ANSWERS TO PRACTICE STRIPS

PRACTICE STRIP #167

Atrial Rhythm:	Regular
Ventricular Rhythm:	Regular
Atrial Rate:	110
Ventricular Rate:	110
P Waves:	Present, one P/complex, uniform
PRI:	.28 seconds
QRS:	.10 seconds
Interpretation:	Sinus Tachycardia with First Degree AV Heart Block

PRACTICE STRIP #168

Atrial Rhythm:	Regular
Ventricular Rhythm:	Regular except for the 9th beat which is early
Atrial Rate:	120
Ventricular Rate:	120
P Waves:	Present, one P/complex except for the 9th beat, uniform
PRI:	.12 seconds
QRS:	.06 seconds except for the 9th complex which is greater than .12 seconds
Interpretation:	Sinus Tachycardia with one PVC

PRACTICE STRIP #169

Atrial Rhythm:	Irregular due to early beats
Ventricular Rhythm:	Irregular due to early beats
Atrial Rate:	60
Ventricular Rate:	100
P Waves:	Present and uniform except for the early beats; every 3rd beat is early
PRI:	.12 seconds
QRS:	.08 seconds except for the early beats which are greater than .12 seconds
Interpretation:	Ventricular Trigeminy

ANSWERS TO PRACTICE STRIPS

PRACTICE STRIP #170

Atrial Rhythm:	Unable to identify P wave
Ventricular Rhythm:	Irregular
Atrial Rate:	Ø
Ventricular Rate:	80
P Waves:	Ø
PRI:	Ø
QRS:	.10 seconds
Interpretation:	Atrial Fibrillation, Controlled

PRACTICE STRIP #171

Atrial Rhythm:	Unable to identify P wave
Ventricular Rhythm:	Irregular
Atrial Rate:	Ø
Ventricular Rate:	160
P Waves:	Ø
PRI:	Ø
QRS:	.08 seconds except for the 14th beat which is .12 seconds
Interpretation:	Atrial Fibrillation, Uncontrolled and one PVC

PRACTICE STRIP #172

Atrial Rhythm:	Unable to identify P wave
Ventricular Rhythm:	Irregular
Atrial Rate:	Ø
Ventricular Rate:	90
P Waves:	Ø
PRI:	Ø
QRS:	.11 seconds except for the 6th, 7th and 9th beats which are greater than .12 seconds
Interpretation:	Atrial Fibrillation, Controlled with Sequential and Multifocal PVC's

ANSWERS TO PRACTICE STRIPS

PRACTICE STRIP #173

Atrial Rhythm:	Regular
Ventricular Rhythm:	Regular
Atrial Rate:	90
Ventricular Rate:	60
P Waves:	Present and uniform, more P's than complexes
PRI:	.16 to .24 seconds, variable with a pattern progressively longer until one P does not conduct to the ventricle
QRS:	.06 seconds
Interpretation:	Mobitz I

PRACTICE STRIP #174

Atrial Rhythm:	Unable to identify P wave
Ventricular Rhythm:	Irregular
Atrial Rate:	0
Ventricular Rate:	50
P Waves:	0
PRI:	0
QRS:	.08 seconds
Interpretation:	Atrial Fibrillation with Bradycardia

PRACTICE STRIP #175

Atrial Rhythm:	Unable to identify P wave
Ventricular Rhythm:	Irregular
Atrial Rate:	0
Ventricular Rate:	70
P Waves:	0
PRI:	0
QRS:	.08 seconds except for the 5th complex which is greater than .12 seconds
Interpretation:	Atrial Fibrillation, Controlled and one PVC

ANSWERS TO PRACTICE STRIPS

PRACTICE STRIP #176

Atrial Rhythm:	Ø
Ventricular Rhythm:	Regular
Atrial Rate:	Ø
Ventricular Rate:	160
P Waves:	Ø
PRI:	Ø
QRS:	Greater than .12 seconds
Interpretation:	Ventricular Tachycardia

PRACTICE STRIP #177

Atrial Rhythm:	Irregular
Ventricular Rhythm:	Irregular
Atrial Rate:	40 (sinus rate 47, junctional rate 37)
Ventricular Rate:	40
P Waves:	Present for first two complexes, absent for last two complexes
PRI:	.12 seconds
QRS:	.06 seconds
Interpretation:	Sinus Bradycardia, Sinus Arrest, Junctional Escape Rhythm with Bradycardia

PRACTICE STRIP #178

Atrial Rhythm:	Unable to ascertain if P's are present
Ventricular Rhythm:	Regular
Atrial Rate:	180 if present
Ventricular Rate:	180
P Waves:	Unable to ascertain if there are P's in the T's
PRI:	Unable to ascertain if there are P's in the T's
QRS:	.08 seconds
Interpretation:	Supraventricular Tachycardia (SVT)

ANSWERS TO PRACTICE STRIPS

PRACTICE STRIP #179

Atrial Rhythm:	Totally chaotic rhythm
Ventricular Rhythm:	Totally chaotic rhythm
Atrial Rate:	0
Ventricular Rate:	0
P Waves:	0
PRI:	0
QRS:	0
Interpretation:	Ventricular Fibrillation

PRACTICE STRIP #180

Atrial Rhythm:	0
Ventricular Rhythm:	Regular
Atrial Rate:	0
Ventricular Rate:	90
P Waves:	0
PRI:	0
QRS:	.12 seconds
Interpretation:	Accelerated Ventricular Rhythm

PRACTICE STRIP #181

Atrial Rhythm:	Regular
Ventricular Rhythm:	Regular except for the 6th beat
Atrial Rate:	107 (Small Box Method)
Ventricular Rate:	110
P Waves:	Present and uniform, one P/complex except for the 6th beat
PRI:	.20 seconds
QRS:	.10 seconds except for the 6th complex which is greater than .12 seconds
Interpretation:	Sinus Tachycardia with one PVC

ANSWERS TO PRACTICE STRIPS

PRACTICE STRIP #182

Atrial Rhythm:	Regular except for the 4th beat
Ventricular Rhythm:	Regular except for the 4th beat
Atrial Rate:	100
Ventricular Rate:	100
P Waves:	Present, one P/complex, uniform except the 4th P is inverted before the complex
PRI:	.16 seconds except the 4th PRI is .12 seconds
QRS:	.08 seconds
Interpretation:	RSR with PAC (the P' is a biphasic P wave-- negative then positive)

PRACTICE STRIP #183

Atrial Rhythm:	Regular except for the 6th and 9th beats
Ventricular Rhythm:	Regular except for the 6th and 9th beats
Atrial Rate:	90
Ventricular Rate:	90
P Waves:	Present, one P/complex, uniform except for 6th and 9th beats which are merged in the T wave
PRI:	.14 seconds
QRS:	.08 seconds
Interpretation:	RSR with two PAC's

PRACTICE STRIP #184

Atrial Rhythm:	Regular
Ventricular Rhythm:	Regular
Atrial Rate:	130
Ventricular Rate:	50
P Waves:	Present and uniform, more P's than complexes
PRI:	.12 seconds
QRS:	.08 seconds
Interpretation:	Mobitz II

ANSWERS TO PRACTICE STRIPS

PRACTICE STRIP #185

Atrial Rhythm:	Regular
Ventricular Rhythm:	Regular
Atrial Rate:	30
Ventricular Rate:	30
P Waves:	Ø
PRI:	Ø
QRS:	Greater than .12 seconds
Interpretation:	Idioventricular Rhythm

PRACTICE STRIP #186

Atrial Rhythm:	Regular
Ventricular Rhythm:	Regular
Atrial Rate:	110
Ventricular Rate:	110
P Waves:	Present, one P/complex, uniform except for artifact
PRI:	.28 seconds, constant
QRS:	.08 seconds
Interpretation:	Sinus Tachycardia with First Degree AV Heart Block

PRACTICE STRIP #187

Atrial Rhythm:	Regular
Ventricular Rhythm:	Irregular
Atrial Rate:	70
Ventricular Rate:	60
P Waves:	Present and uniform
PRI:	Variable with a pattern, .16 to .28 seconds
QRS:	.08 seconds
Interpretation:	Mobitz I

ANSWERS TO PRACTICE STRIPS

PRACTICE STRIP #188

Atrial Rhythm:	∅
Ventricular Rhythm:	Irregular
Atrial Rate:	∅
Ventricular Rate:	160
P Waves:	∅
PRI:	∅
QRS:	Greater than .12 seconds
Interpretation:	Ventricular Tachycardia

PRACTICE STRIP #189

Atrial Rhythm:	Unable to identify P wave
Ventricular Rhythm:	Irregular
Atrial Rate:	∅
Ventricular Rate:	90
P Waves:	∅
PRI:	∅
QRS:	.10 seconds
Interpretation:	Atrial Fibrillation, Controlled

PRACTICE STRIP #190

Atrial Rhythm:	Regular
Ventricular Rhythm:	Regular
Atrial Rate:	90
Ventricular Rate:	50
P Waves:	Present and uniform, more P's than complexes
PRI:	.18 seconds, constant
QRS:	.08 seconds
Interpretation:	Mobitz II

ANSWERS TO PRACTICE STRIPS

PRACTICE STRIP #191

Atrial Rhythm:	Regular
Ventricular Rhythm:	Irregular
Atrial Rate:	90
Ventricular Rate:	60
P Waves:	Present and uniform, more P's than complexes
PRI:	Variable with a pattern, .12 to .24 seconds
QRS:	.08 seconds
Interpretation:	Mobitz I

PRACTICE STRIP #192

Atrial Rhythm:	Regular
Ventricular Rhythm:	Regular
Atrial Rate:	50
Ventricular Rate:	50
P Waves:	Present, one P/complex, uniform
PRI:	.32 seconds, constant
QRS:	.08 seconds
Interpretation:	Sinus Bradycardia with First Degree AV Heart Block

PRACTICE STRIP #193

Atrial Rhythm:	Regular
Ventricular Rhythm:	Regular
Atrial Rate:	70
Ventricular Rate:	70
P Waves:	Present, one P/complex, uniform
PRI:	.24 seconds, constant
QRS:	.14 seconds
Interpretation:	RSR with First Degree A-V Heart Block and Aberrant Ventricular Conduction

ANSWERS TO PRACTICE STRIPS
PRACTICE STRIP #194

Atrial Rhythm:	Unable to identify P wave
Ventricular Rhythm:	Irregular
Atrial Rate:	0
Ventricular Rate:	150
P Waves:	0
PRI:	0
QRS:	.08 seconds except for the two bizarre beats
Interpretation:	Atrial Fibrillation, Uncontrolled, and two PVC's

PRACTICE STRIP #195

Atrial Rhythm:	Regular
Ventricular Rhythm:	Irregular
Atrial Rate:	80
Ventricular Rate:	70
P Waves:	Present, more P's than complexes
PRI:	Variable with a pattern
QRS:	.06 seconds except for the bizarre 4th beat
Interpretation:	Mobitz I with one PVC

PRACTICE STRIP #196

Atrial Rhythm:	Regular
Ventricular Rhythm:	Regular
Atrial Rate:	140
Ventricular Rate:	60
P Waves:	Present, one P/complex except for the bizarre beat
PRI:	.12 seconds
QRS:	.06 seconds except for the bizarre 6th beat which is also early
Interpretation:	Mobitz II with one PVC

CHAPTER 9: BASIC ARRHYTHMIA ECG REVIEW

This chapter reviews all the characteristics of the Basic Arrhythmias. The causes, significance and interventions are included.

An arrhythmia is significant **if:**

1.   It decreases Cardiac Output

     You will recall that Cardiac Output is the amount of blood the heart ejects in one minute.

     Cardiac Output = Stroke Volume times Heart Rate

     Stroke Volume is the amount of blood the heart ejects with each systole.

QUESTION

The average Stroke Volume is 70 ml and the average Heart Rate is 70 BPM (beats per minute) for an adult. Calculate an average Cardiac Output based on this example.

ANSWER

70 ml X 70 BPM = 4900 ml. The normal Cardiac Output for the adult is 4 to 6 liters per minute.

QUESTION

What effect would a decrease in heart rate (with no change in Stroke Volume) have upon the Cardiac Output?

ANSWER

A decrease in heart rate without an increase in stroke volume decreases Cardiac Output. One significant thing about any bradycardia is that it DECREASES CARDIAC OUTPUT.

Tachycardias tend to increase Cardiac Output according to the formula. However, tachycardias ONLY increase Cardiac Output up to a point. As the heart rate increases the time of diastole is forced to decrease. A point is reached in tachycardias where the time of diastole is so short there is not adequate time on diastole for filling.

QUESTION

What is one significant thing about tachycardias?

ANSWER

Tachycardias may DECREASE CARDIAC OUTPUT.

Consider next the coronary arteries. Pretend your hand is your heart and your fingerprints on the palm of the hand are your coronary arteries. Squeeze your hand, making a fist, similar to the heart pumping--open it, squeeze it. Look at what is happening to the coronary arteries and answer the next question.

QUESTION

When do the coronary arteries receive perfusion, on systole or on diastole?

ANSWER

The coronary arteries receive their perfusion on diastole. On systole they are being squeezed shut by the pumping action of the myocardium.

QUESTION

Name another significant thing about tachycardias.

ANSWER

Tachycardias decrease coronary artery perfusion. Tachycardias increase the demands upon the heart by causing it to beat faster at the same time it is decreasing coronary artery perfusion.

An arrhythmia is significant if: (Cont'd)

2.   Some categories of arrhythmias are significant because they signal irritability of the myocardium. Premature ectopic beats are examples of this.

3.   Some arrhythmias are significant because they may be the forerunner of more serious arrhythmias. An example is first degree A-V heart block, which usually does not compromise cardiac output, but it may deteriorate into a higher degree of block.

4. Arrhythmias that originate in the ventricle are also significant. Consider the anatomy of the conduction system of the heart.

QUESTION

The sinus node is the normal pacemaker of the heart. If the sinus node fails, can another pacemaker take over?

ANSWER

Yes, the atria or another ectopic can take over control of the heart.

QUESTION

If the sinus node fails and the atria fail, can another pacemaker take over?

ANSWER

Yes, the A-V junction can take over control of the heart.

QUESTION

If the sinus node fails and the atria fail and the A-V junction fails, can another pacemaker take over?

ANSWER

Yes, the ventricles can take over control of the heart.

QUESTION

If the sinus node fails and the atria fail and the A-V junction fails and the ventricles fail, can another pacemaker take over?

ANSWER

No, the ventricles are the last escape pacemaker of the heart.

On pages 257 through 284 of this Manual, review the ECG characteristics, causes, significance and interventions of the Basic Arrhythmias. Remember, arrhythmias should not be treated unless the patient is symptomatic. ARRHYTHMIAS ARE NOT TREATED--PATIENTS ARE TREATED!!

NORMAL SINUS RHYTHM

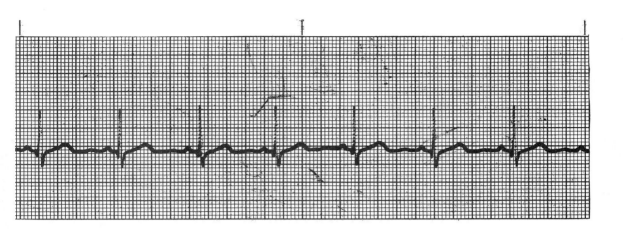

RHYTHM:	ATRIAL: Regular VENTRICULAR: Regular
RATE:	ATRIAL: 60 to 100 VENTRICULAR: 60 to 100
P WAVES:	Present and uniform, one per complex
PRI:	.12 to .20 seconds; constant
QRS:	Less than .12 seconds .12 seconds or more if conduction is aberrant
CAUSES:	Normal
SIGNIFICANCE:	None
INTERVENTION:	Observe the patient

*Normal Sinus Rhythm

SINUS BRADYCARDIA

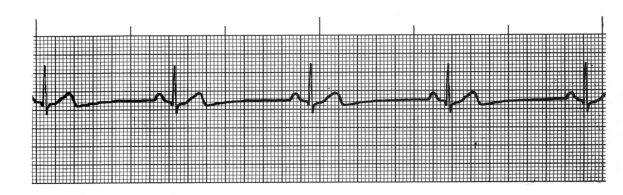

RHYTHM:	ATRIAL: Regular VENTRICULAR: Regular
RATE:	ATRIAL: Less than 60 VENTRICULAR: Less than 60
P WAVES:	Present and uniform, one per complex
PRI:	.12 to .20 seconds; constant
QRS:	Less than .12 seconds .12 seconds or more if conduction is aberrant
CAUSES:	Athletic heart, increased vagal tone, increased intracranial pressure, decreased metabolic needs (e.g. sleep), acute myocardial infarction, digitalis administration, hypothyroidism, etc.
SIGNIFICANCE:	May decrease cardiac output
INTERVENTION:	Atropine, rarely an artificial pacemaker may be necessary. Isoproterenol may be required as a temporizing therapy.

SINUS TACHYCARDIA

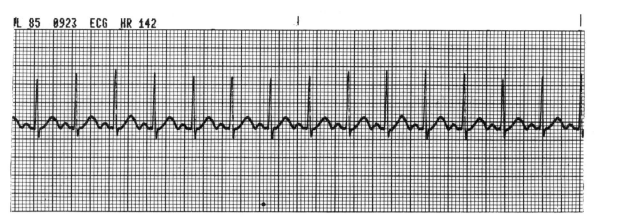

ML 85 0923 ECG HR 142

RHYTHM: ATRIAL: Regular
VENTRICULAR: Regular

RATE: ATRIAL: 101 to 160
VENTRICULAR: 101 to 160

P WAVES: Present and uniform, one per complex

PRI: .12 to .20 seconds; constant

QRS: Less than .12 seconds
.12 seconds or more if conduction is aberrant

CAUSES: Heart failure, infections, anemia, hypoxia, thyrotoxicosis, sympathetic stimulation, exercise, exertions, digitalis toxicity, etc. Drugs such as Aminophylline, Atropine, Isoproternenol, Epinephrine.

SIGNIFICANCE: -May decrease cardiac output
-Increases work load of the heart

INTERVENTION: Find and treat the cause

SINUS ARRHYTHMIA

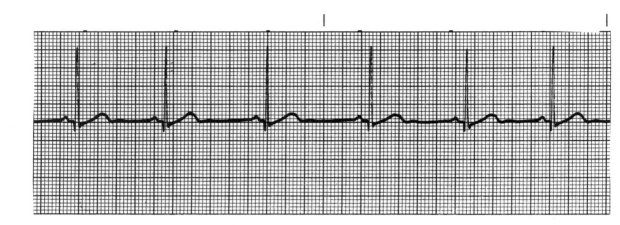

RHYTHM:	ATRIAL: Irregular VENTRICULAR: Irregular
RATE:	ATRIAL: 60 to 100 VENTRICULAR: 60 to 100
P WAVES:	Present and uniform, one per complex
PRI:	.12 to .20 seconds; constant
QRS:	Less than .12 seconds .12 seconds or more if conduction is aberrant
CAUSES:	This arrhythmia is usually due to the pressure changes on inspiration and expiration; the arrhythmia will wax and wane with respiration. May be caused by digitalis or quinidine administration (rare).
SIGNIFICANCE:	Insignificant, unless caused by digitalis or quinidine toxicity
INTERVENTION:	Observe the patient; discontinue toxic drugs

SINUS ARREST

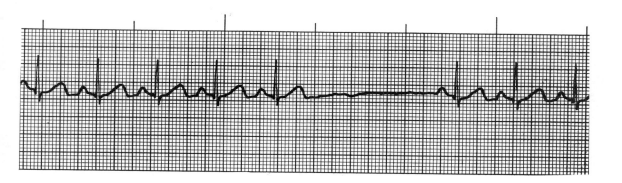

RHYTHM: ATRIAL: Irregular due to the arrest
VENTRICULAR: Irregular due to the arrest

RATE: ATRIAL: Slowed due to the arrest
VENTRICULAR: Slowed due to the arrest

P WAVES: Absent during the arrest

PRI: No P wave or complex during the arrest; therefore, no
PRI

QRS: Absent during the arrest; an ectopic pacemaker may
escape to depolarize the ventricle.

CAUSES: Increased vagal tone, acute myocardial infarction
(inferior wall), digitalis and quinidine toxicity,
administration of parasympathomimetic drugs.

INTERVENTION: Atropine, pacemaker--discontinue toxic drugs.
Isoproterenol may be required as temporizing therapy.

PREMATURE ATRIAL CONTRACTION (PAC)

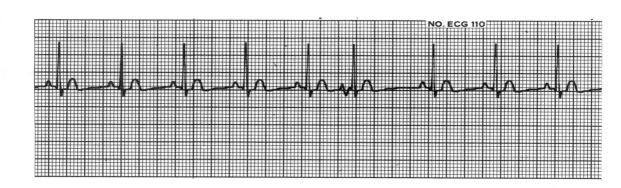

NO. ECG 110

RHYTHM:	ATRIAL: Irregular due to the PAC VENTRICULAR: Irregular due to the PAC
RATE:	ATRIAL: May be increased due to the PAC's VENTRICULAR: May be changed due to the PAC
P WAVES:	P' (P wave of the PAC) is early and looks different than the sinus P wave
PRI:	P'RI will be the same as or longer than the PRI of the sinus beat
QRS:	-Less than .12 seconds if conduction is normal -.12 seconds or more if conduction is aberrant -Absent if the PAC is nonconducted
CAUSES:	Organic heart disease, thyrotoxicosis, digitalis intoxication stress, nicotine, alcohol, caffeine, etc.
SIGNIFICANCE:	5 PAC's in a row constitute a run of atrial tachycardia (PAT)
INTERVENTION:	- Remove the cause -Usually are not treated unless frequent or cause PAT -Suppressant drugs include digitalis, quinidine, procainamide propranalol

PAROXYSMAL ATRIAL TACHYCARDIA (PAT)

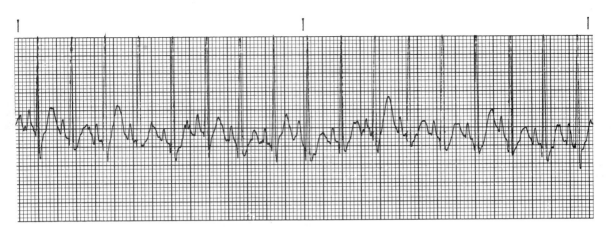

RHYTHM: ATRIAL: Regular
                VENTRICULAR: Regular

RATE: ATRIAL: 150 to 250
                VENTRICULAR: Equal to or less than the Atrial Rate

P WAVES: Present and uniform but may be difficult to see

PRI: .12 to .20 seconds; constant
                -All P's may not conduct

QRS: Less than .12 seconds
                .12 seconds or more if conduction is aberrant

CAUSES: Organic heart disease, thyrotoxicosis, digitalis
                intoxication, stress, nicotine, alcohol, caffeine, etc.

SIGNIFICANCE: Rapid ventricular rate may decrease cardiac
                output and   compromise the patient

INTERVENTION: Carotid massage or other vagal stimuli, oxygen, digitalis,
                quinidine, calcium blockers (Verapamil), propranalol,
                cardioversion, atrial pacemaker

ATRIAL FLUTTER

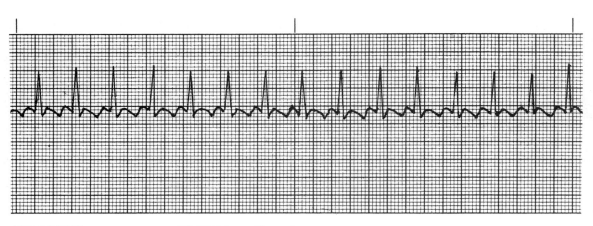

RHYTHM: ATRIAL: Regular
VENTRICULAR: Regular or irregular*

RATE: ATRIAL: 250 to 350
VENTRICULAR: Depends on conduction which may
be 1:1, 2:1, 3:1, 4:1, (up to 8:1)

P WAVES: Flutter waves with a sawtooth appearance (F waves);
these Flutter waves are constant

PRI: Unable to measure a PRI as there is no P wave

QRS: Less than .12 seconds
.12 seconds or more if conduction is aberrant

CAUSES: Organic heart disease--such as rheumatic heart
disease, digitalis intoxication (rare)

SIGNIFICANCE: -Rapid ventricular rate may decrease cardiac output
-Frequently precedes atrial fibrillation

INTERVENTION: Digitalis, quinidine, calcium blockers (e.g. Verapamil),
propranalol, cardioversion, atrial pacemaker
If the ventricular rate is slow, suspect digitalis toxicity

*Conduction may be variable resulting in irregular ventricular rhythm

ATRIAL FIBRILLATION

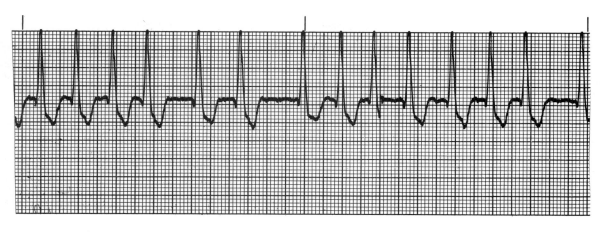

RHYTHM:	ATRIAL: Irregular, unable to identify P wave VENTRICULAR: Irregular
RATE:	ATRIAL: Rapid (unable to count on ECG) VENTRICULAR: Controlled = less than 100 per minute Uncontrolled = 100 or more per minute
P WAVES:	Uneven and irregular atrial activity results in a fibrillatory wave (f wave); f wave may be coarse, fine or isoelectric
PRI:	Unable to measure as there are no P waves
QRS:	Less than .12 seconds .12 seconds or more if conduction is aberrant
CAUSES:	Organic heart disease such as mitral valve disease, digitalis intoxication.
SIGNIFICANCE:	-Rapid ventricular rate may decrease cardiac output -Decreased cardiac output due to loss of synchronization between the atria and ventricles -Stasis of blood may cause pulmonary or cerebral embolism
INTERVENTION:	-Digitalis, quindine, calcium blockers (e.g., Verapamil), cardioversion, atrial pacemaker if needed to slow the ventricular rate. -Monitor the patient for changes in respiratory or neurologic status -If the ventricular rate is slow, suspect digitalis toxicity.

PREMATURE JUNCTIONAL CONTRACTION (PJC)

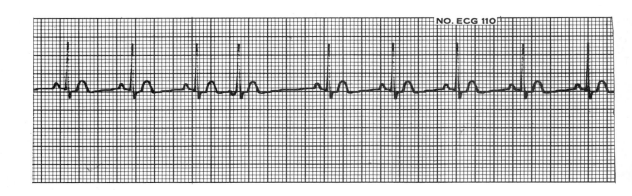

NO. ECG 110

RHYTHM:	ATRIAL: Irregular due to the PJC VENTRICULAR: Irregular due to the PJC
RATE:	ATRIAL: May be increased due to the PJC VENTRICULAR: May be increased due to the PJC
P WAVES:	P wave of the PJC will be inverted before or after the complex or it will be absent
PRI:	If present will be .12 seconds or less
QRS:	Less than .12 seconds .12 seconds or more if conduction is aberrant
CAUSES:	Ischemic and organic heart disease
SIGNIFICANCE:	May be warning of myocardial irritability
INTERVENTION:	-Usually not treated unless frequent (more than 5 per minute) -Suppressant drugs include digitalis, quinidine, procainamide, Verapamil

JUNCTIONAL TACHYCARDIA

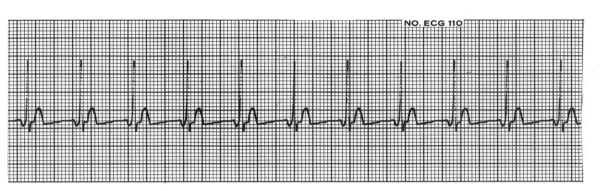

NO. ECG 110

RHYTHM: ATRIAL: Regular
VENTRICULAR: Regular

RATE: ATRIAL: 101 to 200
VENTRICULAR: 101 to 200

P WAVES: Inverted before or after the complex or absent

PRI: .12 seconds or less when present

QRS: Less than .12 seconds
.12 seconds or more if conduction is aberrant

CAUSES: Coronary artery disease, cardiac valve disease, heart trauma, heart surgery, digitalis intoxication

SIGNIFICANCE: -The irritable junctional ectopic has taken over as the pacemaker of the heart
-Rapid ventricular rate may decrease cardiac output
-Loss of synchronization between the atria and ventricles may cause decreased cardiac output

INTERVENTION: Suppressant drugs include digitalis, quinidine, procainamide, Verapamil, Lidocaine

JUNCTIONAL ESCAPE BEAT

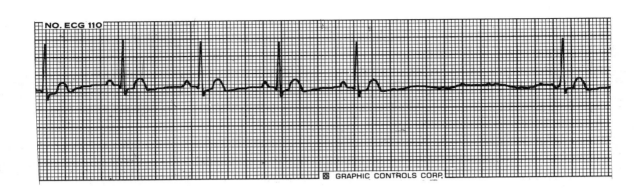

RHYTHM: ATRIAL: Irregular due to the Sinus Arrest
VENTRICULAR: Irregular due to the Sinus Arrest

RATE: ATRIAL: Slowed due to the Sinus Arrest
VENTRICULAR: Slowed due to the Sinus Arrest

P WAVES: P wave of the Junctional Escape Beat will be inverted before or after the complex or it will be absent

PRI: The PRI of the Junctional Escape Beats will be .12 seconds or less when present. The PRI of the sinus beats is .12 to .20 seconds

QRS: Less than .12 seconds

CAUSES: The Junctional Ectopic escapes due to the arrest of the sinus node

SIGNIFICANCE: Failure of the sinus node

INTERVENTION: Therapy may be indicated for the sinus node arrest -- Atropine artificial pacemaker

JUNCTIONAL ESCAPE RHYTHM

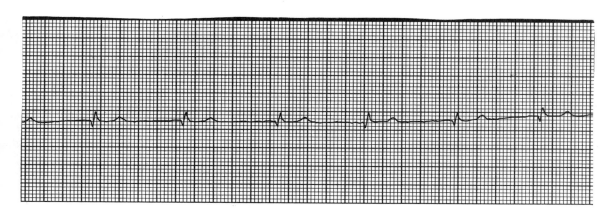

RHYTHM: ATRIAL: Regular
                     VENTRICULAR: Regular

RATE: ATRIAL: 40 to 60
                     VENTRICULAR: 40 to 60

P WAVES: Inverted before or after the complex or absent

PRI: .12 seconds or less when present

QRS: Less than .12 seconds

CAUSES: -Failure of the sinus node
                     -The sinus node has arrested allowing this ectopic to escape
                     -The junctional ectopic is pacing the heart at its inherent rate

SIGNIFICANCE: May cause decreased cardiac output due to the slow ventricular
                     rate

INTERVENTION: Atropine, artificial pacemaker may be necessary

JUNCTIONAL BRADYCARDIA

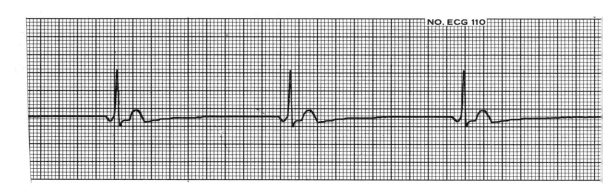

NO. ECG 110

RHYTHM: ATRIAL: Regular
                             VENTRICULAR: Regular

RATE: ATRIAL: Less than 40
                             VENTRICULAR: Less than 40

P WAVES: Inverted before or after the complex or absent

PRI: .12 seconds or less when present

QRS: Less than .12 seconds

CAUSES: -Failure of the sinus node
                             -The sinus node has arrested allowing this ectopic to
                               escape
                             -The junctional ectopic is pacing the heart at less
                               than its inherent rate

SIGNIFICANCE: Decreased cardiac output due to slow ventricular rate

INTERVENTION: Treatment is aimed at increasing the rate; Atropine, artificial pacemaker, Isoproterenol as a temporizing therapy

ACCELERATED JUNCTIONAL RHYTHM

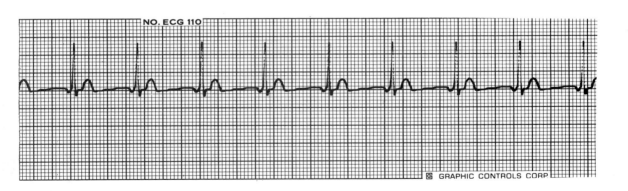

NO. ECG 110

Ⓖ GRAPHIC CONTROLS CORP

RHYTHM: ATRIAL: Regular
VENTRICULAR: Regular

RATE: ATRIAL: 61 to 100
VENTRICULAR: 61 to 100

P WAVES: Inverted before or after the complex or absent

PRI: .12 seconds or less when present

QRS: Less than .12 seconds

CAUSES: The junctional ectopic is pacing the heart faster than its inherent rate, but less than a tachycardia

SIGNIFICANCE: Does not usually compromise the patient

INTERVENTION: Observe the patient

WANDERING PACEMAKER

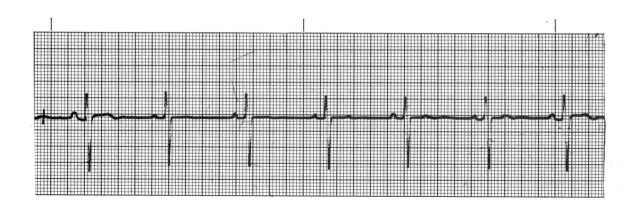

RHYTHM: ATRIAL: Regular or slightly irregular
                                   VENTRICULAR: Regular or slightly irregular

RATE: ATRIAL: 60 to 100
                                   VENTRICULAR: 60 to 100

P WAVES: Three or more different configurations in one lead.
Some may be inverted or absent depending on pacemaker site

PRI: Less than .12 seconds when present

QRS: Less than .12 seconds

CAUSES: The pacemaker site wanders among the sinus node, atrial and junctional ectopics

SIGNIFICANCE: Although some beats originate from ectopics sites, the heart rate is usually normal

INTERVENTION: Observe the patient

SUPRAVENTRICULAR TACHYCARDIA

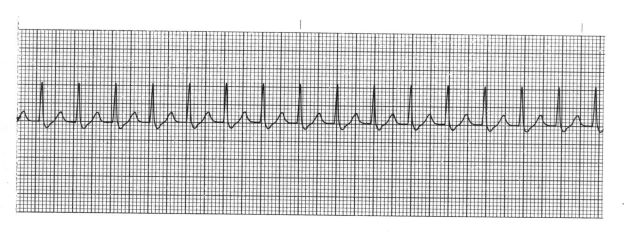

RHYTHM:	ATRIAL: Regular VENTRICULAR: Regular
RATE:	ATRIAL: Over 140 VENTRICULAR: Over 140
P WAVES:	May or may not be present; may be difficult to discern
PRI:	.12 to .20 seconds if present
QRS:	Less than .12 seconds
CAUSES:	Same as the causes of Sinus Tachycardia, Atrial Tachycardias and Junctional Tachycardia
INTERVENTION:	Carotid massage may be used to convert the arrhythmia or to help diagnose it. Rest, oxygen, and sedation. Suppressant drugs include digitalis, quinidine, Verapamil, procainamide

FIRST DEGREE A-V HEART BLOCK

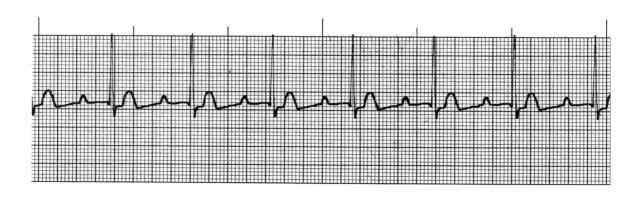

RHYTHM: ATRIAL: May be regular or irregular
                          VENTRICULAR: May be regular or irregular

RATE: ATRIAL: May be slow, fast or normal
                          VENTRICULAR: May be slow, fast or normal

P WAVES: Present and uniform, one per complex

PRI: Greater than .20 seconds, constant

QRS: Less than .12 seconds

CAUSES: Acute myocardial infarction, drugs such as digitalis and procainamide, hyperkalemia; may be congenital

INTERVENTION: -Discontinue toxic drugs
-Treat hyperkalemia
-Observe patient for the development of a higher degree of block

SECOND DEGREE A-V HEART BLOCK TYPE I*

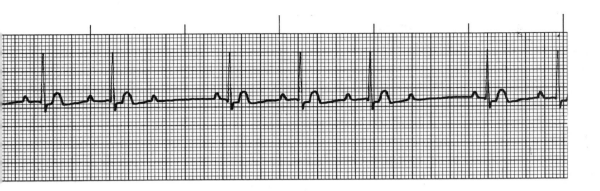

RHYTHM: ATRIAL: Regular or irregular
         VENTRICULAR: Irregular

RATE: ATRIAL: Usually normal
         VENTRICULAR: Less than the Atrial Rate

P WAVES: Present and uniform, more P's than complexes

PRI: Progressively longer until one does not conduct, then
         the cycle starts over

QRS: Less than .12 seconds

CAUSES: Acute myocardial infarction; drugs; such as
         digitalis and procainamide; hyperkalemia; may be
         congenital

SIGNIFICANCE: This type of block is usually transient but it may
         progress to a higher degree of block

INTERVENTION: -Discontinue toxic drugs
         -Treat hyperkalemia
         -Observe patient for the development of a higher degree
         of block

*Wenckebach, Mobitz I

SECOND DEGREE A-V HEART BLOCK TYPE II*

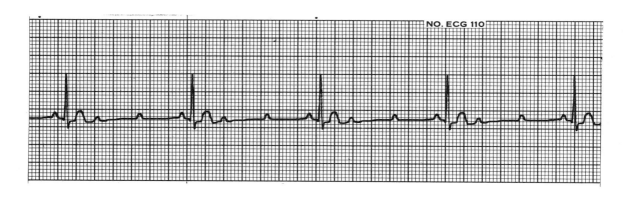

NO. ECG 110

RHYTHM:	ATRIAL: Regular or irregular VENTRICULAR: Regular or irregular
RATE:	ATRIAL: Usually normal VENTRICULAR: Less than the Atrial Rate
P WAVES:	Present and uniform, more P's than complexes
PRI:	May be normal or prolonged; PRI is constant for those P's that do conduct
QRS:	May be normal but a wide complex is not unusual with this type of A-V block
CAUSES:	Acute myocardial infarction; drugs (e.g. digitalis and procainamide); hyperkalemia; may be congenital
SIGNIFICANCE:	-Decreased cardiac output due to slow ventricular rate -This type of A-V block frequently precedes sudden Complete Heart Block
INTERVENTION:	-Definitive therapy is usually a pacemaker -Drug therapy may include Atropine and Isoproterenol -Isoproterenol may be required as temporizing therapy

*Mobitz II

THIRD DEGREE A-V HEART BLOCK*

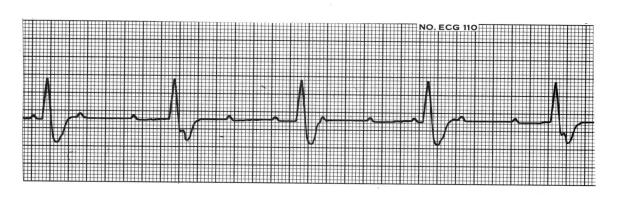

NO. ECG 110

RHYTHM:	ATRIAL: That of the prevailing atrial rhythm VENTRICULAR: Regular
RATE:	ATRIAL: May be slow, normal or rapid VENTRICULAR: Slow
P WAVES:	Present, but may be lost in or distorted by the complex
PRI:	Variable. The P's are unrelated to the complex
QRS:	May be normal or wider than normal
CAUSES:	Acute myocardial infarction; drugs (e.g. digitalis and procainamide); hyperkalemia; may be congenital
SIGNIFICANCE:	-Decreased cardiac output due to slow ventricular rate
INTERVENTION:	-Definitive therapy is usually a pacemaker -Drug therapy may include Atropine and Isoproterenol as temporizing therapy

*Complete Heart Block

PREMATURE VENTRICULAR CONTRACTIONS

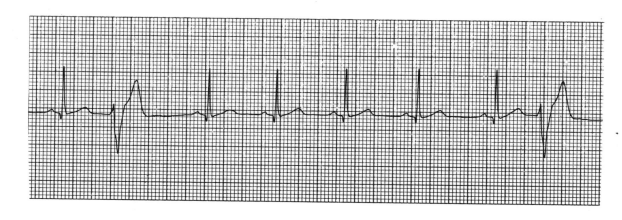

RHYTHM: ATRIAL: P wave is usually lost in the PVC
VENTRICULAR: Irregular due to the PVC

RATE: ATRIAL: Unchanged
VENTRICULAR: May be increased due to the PVC

P WAVES: Usually lost in the PVC

PRI: Not measured for the PVC

QRS: The complex of the PVC is .12 seconds or greater
with bizarre appearance — ST segment and T wave are
in the opposite direction to the main part of the complex

CAUSES: Nicotine, caffeine, stress, hypoxia, heart disease,
electrolyte imbalance, digitalis intoxication

SIGNIFICANCE: -Frequent (6 or more per minute usually require
intervention)
-Multifocal or paired indicate increased myocardial
irritability
-Three or more PVC's in a row constitute a run of
Ventricular Tachycardia

INTERVENTION: -Remove cause of PVC's
-Oxygen
-Lidocaine, procainamide, Bretylium
-Atropine if the PVC's are due to hypoxia caused by
bradycardia

VENTRICULAR TACHYCARDIA

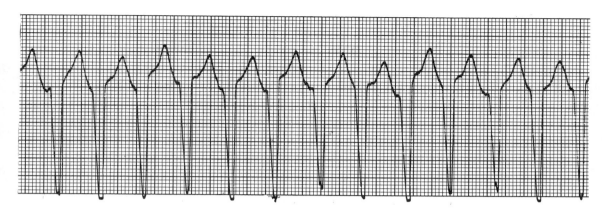

RHYTHM: ATRIAL: There usually are no P waves
                    VENTRICULAR: Regular

RATE: ATRIAL: There usually are no P waves
                    VENTRICULAR: 101 to 250*

P WAVES: Usually not visible

PRI: Do not measure

QRS: .12 seconds or greater, bizarre appearance

CAUSES: Nicotine, caffeine, stress, hypoxia, heart disease,
                    electrolyte imbalance, digitalis intoxication

SIGNIFICANCE: Decreased cardiac output due to tachycardia and the
                    loss of A-V synchronization

INTERVENTION: Lidocaine, procainamide, Bretylium, cardioversion/
                    defibrillation

*Ventricular rate more than 250 is called Ventricular Flutter

VENTRICULAR ESCAPE BEAT

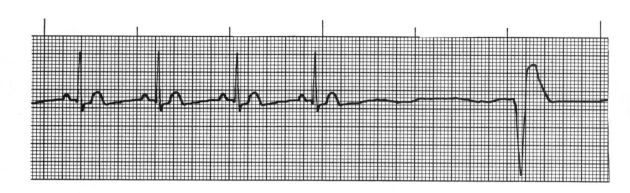

RHYTHM: ATRIAL: Irregular due to the Sinus Arrest
                     VENTRICULAR: Irregular due to the Sinus Arrest

RATE: ATRIAL: Irregular due to the Sinus Arrest
                     VENTRICULAR: Irregular due to the Sinus Arrest

P WAVES: The Ventricular Escape Beat will not have a P wave

PRI: The Ventricular Escape Beat will not have a P wave and
                     therefore no PRI

QRS: The Ventricular Escape Beat will be .12 seconds or
                     greater in duration with bizarre appearance

CAUSES: The ventricular ectopic escapes due to failure
                     of higher pacemakers

SIGNIFICANCE: Failure of the higher pacemakers (Sinus, atrial and junctional

INTERVENTION: Therapy may be indicated for the arrest of the higher
                     pacemakers--Atropine, artificial pacemaker
                     -Isoproterenol may be required as a temporizing therapy

IDIOVENTRICULAR RHYTHM

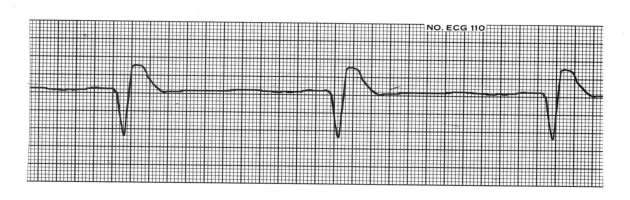

NO. ECG 110

RHYTHM: ATRIAL: There are no P waves
VENTRICULAR: Regular

RATE: ATRIAL: There are no P waves
VENTRICULAR: 40 or less

P WAVES: Usually not seen

PRI: There is no PRI

QRS: .12 seconds or greater with bizarre appearance

CAUSES: Failure of higher pacemakers allow this ventricular ectopic to escape

SIGNIFICANCE: Decreased cardiac output due to bradycardia

INTERVENTION: -Atropine, artificial pacemaker
-Isoproterenol may be required as a temporizing therapy
-May require CPR

ACCELERATED VENTRICULAR RHYTHM

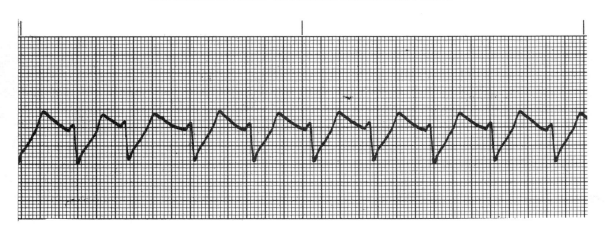

RHYTHM: ATRIAL: There are no P waves
                     VENTRICULAR: Regular

RATE: ATRIAL: There are no P waves
                     VENTRICULAR: 41 to 100

P WAVES: Usually not seen

PRI: There is no PRI

QRS: .12 seconds or greater with bizarre appearance

CAUSES: Failure of higher pacemakers

SIGNIFICANCE: May be a relatively benign arrhythmia or may
                     compromise the patient and require intervention

INTERVENTION: Observe the patient. If cardiac output is impaired
                     due to bradycardia then the atrial rate should be
                     accelerated with Atropine; if this fails, then an artificial
                     atrial pacemaker may be used so that this ventricular
                     ectopic has no chance to reassert itself.

VENTRICULAR FIBRILLATION

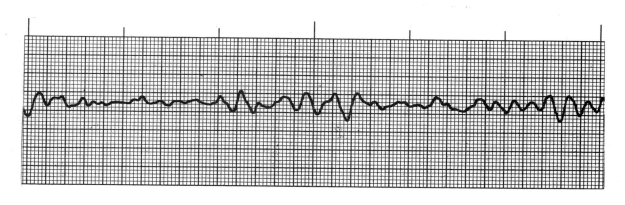

RHYTHM: ATRIAL: There are no P waves
              VENTRICULAR: Totally chaotic

RATE: ATRIAL: There are no P waves
              VENTRICULAR: There are no complexes

P WAVES: None seen

PRI: There is no PRI

QRS: Totally chaotic baseline

CAUSES: The patient is clinically dead

SIGNIFICANCE: There is no cardiac output and the patient is clinically
              dead. CPR must be started immediately to prevent
              biological death

INTERVENTION: CPR and use of CPR drugs, such as, oxygen,
              epinephrine, Lidocaine, Bretylium and sodium
              Definitive treatment is defibrillation.
              bicarbonate.

ASYSTOLE

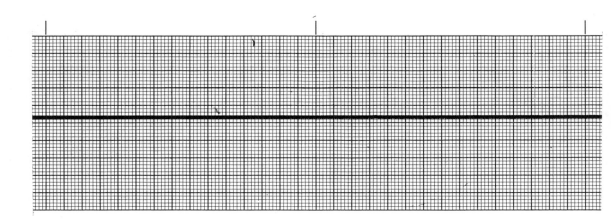

RHYTHM:	ATRIAL: There is no atrial activity VENTRICULAR: There is no ventricular activity
RATE:	ATRIAL: Ø VENTRICULAR: Ø
P WAVES:	No P waves, only a straight line
PRI:	Ø
QRS:	No complex, only a straight line
CAUSES:	The patient is clinically dead
SIGNIFICANCE:	There is no cardiac output and the patient is clinically dead. CPR must be started immediately to prevent biological death
INTERVENTION:	CPR, oxygen, epinephrine, isoproterenol, artificial pacemaker

CHAPTER 10

FINAL EXAMINATION

INSTRUCTIONS: Select the best answer for the following multiple choice questions. Passing score is 75% or better (each question worth 2½ points)

1.

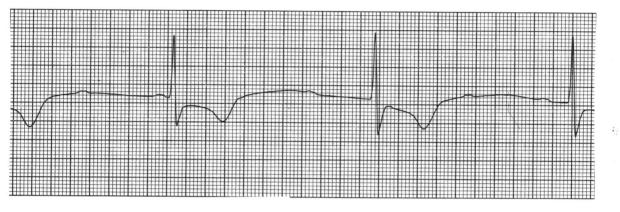

    Interpretation of the above strip is:

        a. Atrial Bradycardia
        b. Junctional Escape Rhythm
        c. Complete Heart Block
        d. Sinus Bradycardia

2. An appropriate intervention for the above strip is:

        a. Verapamil
        b. Carotid massage
        c. Pacemaker
        d. Cardioversion

-285-

3.

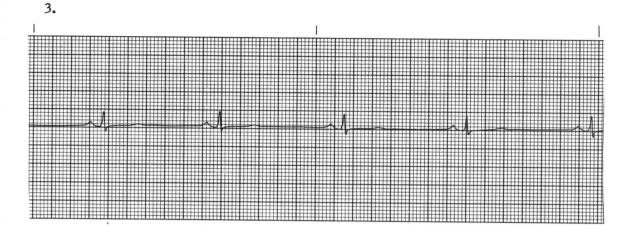

Interpretation of the above strip is:

    a.   Mobitz I
    b.   Sinus Bradycardia
    c.   Atrial Bradycardia
    d.   First Degree A-V Heart Block

4.   An appropriate intervention for the above strip is:

    a.   Verapamil
    b.   Cardioversion
    c.   Procainamide
    d.   Atropine

5.

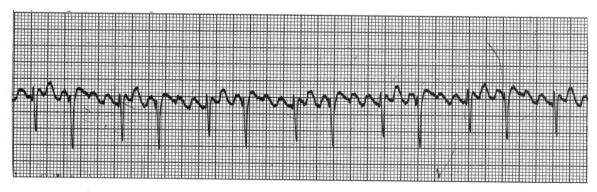

Interpretation of the above strip is:

    a.   Atrial Flutter
    b.   Variable Conduction
    c.   Tachycardia
    d.   Uncontrolled Atrial Fibrillation
    e.   a, b and c

6.   An appropriate intervention for the previous strip is:

        a.   Observe the patient
        b.   Atropine
        c.   Find and treat the cause
        d.   Digoxin

7.

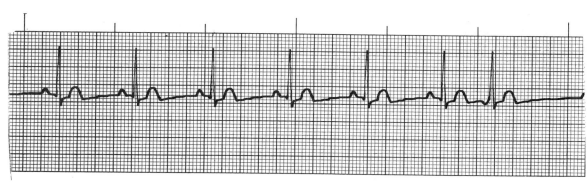

Interpretation of the above strip is:

        a.   RSR with PJC
        b.   Mobitz I
        c.   Sinus Arrhythmia
        d.   RSR with PAC

8.   An appropriate intervention for the above strip is:

        a.   Observe the patient
        b.   Atropine
        c.   Epinephrine
        d.   Isoproterenol

9.

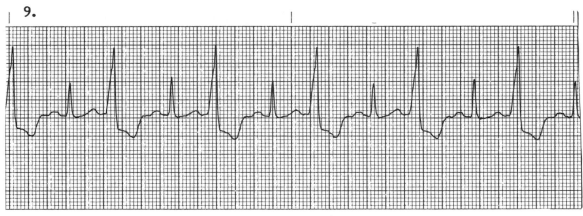

Interpretation of the above strip is:

      a.   Atrial Bigeminy
      b.   Sinus Arrhythmia
      c.   Mobitz II
      d.   Ventricular Bigeminy

10.   An appropriate intervention for the above strip is:

      a.   Digitalis
      b.   Epinephrine
      c.   Lidocaine
      d.   Carotid massage

11.

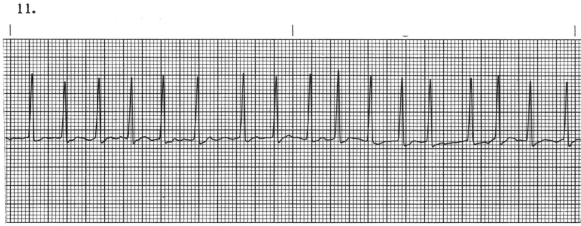

Interpretation of the above strip is:

      a.   Junctional Tachycardia
      b.   Sinus Tachycardia
      c.   Controlled Atrial Fibrillation
      d.   Uncontrolled Atrial Fibrillation

12. An appropriate intervention for the previous strip is:

    a. Digoxin
    b. Atropine
    c. Bretylium
    d. Calcium Chloride

13.

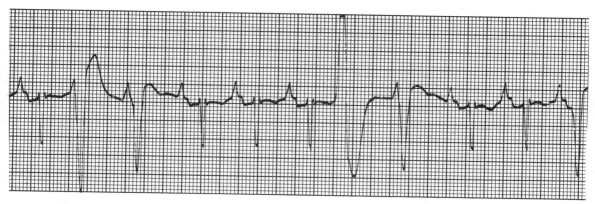

Interpretation of the above strip is:

    a. RSR
    b. PVC
    c. Multifocal and Sequential
    d. First Degree A-V Heart Block
    e. All of the above

14. An appropriate intervention for the above strip is:

    a. °Lidocaine
    b. Calcium Chloride
    c. Epinephrine
    d. Isoproterenol

15.

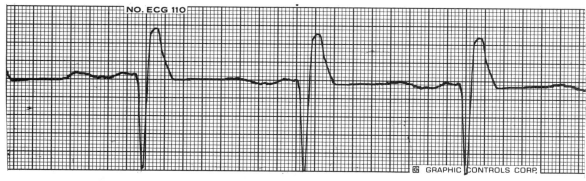

Interpretation of the above strip is:

   a.   Idioventricular Rhythm
   b.   Complete Heart Block
   c.   Sinus Bradycardia
   d.   Accelerated Junctional Rhythm

16.   An appropriate intervention for the above strip is:

   a.   Quinidine
   b.   Diphenylhydantoin
   c.   Atropine
   d.   Carotid massage

17.

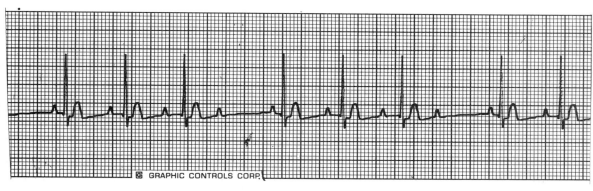

Interpretation of the above strip is:

   a.   Mobitz I
   b.   Mobitz II
   c.   Complete Heart Block
   d.   Sinus Arrhythmia
   e.   RSR with several PAC's

18. An appropriate intervention for the previous strip is:

    a. Sodium Bicarbonate
    b. Pacemaker
    c. Digitalis
    d. Observe the patient

19.

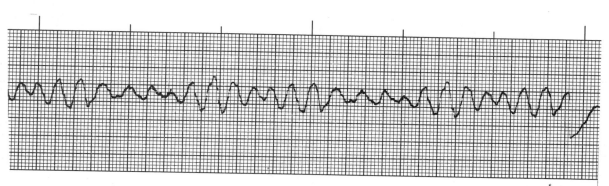

    Interpretation of the above strip is:

    a. Atrial Flutter, Nonconducted
    b. Ventricular Fibrillation
    c. Sinus Tachycardia
    d. Atrial Fibrillation, Nonconducted

20. An appropriate intervention for the above strip is:

    a. CPR
    b. Digitalis
    c. Find and treat the cause
    d. Verapamil

21.

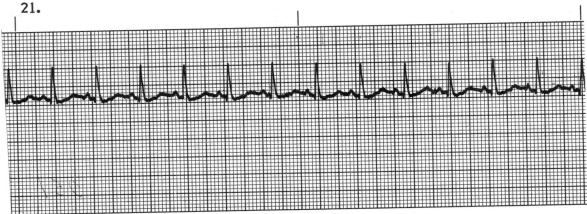

Interpretation of the above strip is:

    a.   Atrial Flutter 2:1
    b.   Sinus Tachycardia
    c.   First Degree AV Block
    d.   RSR
    e.   c and d

22.   An appropriate intervention for the above strip is:

    a.   Cardioversion
    b.   Verapamil
    c.   Observe for a higher degree of A-V Block
    d.   Find and treat the cause

23.

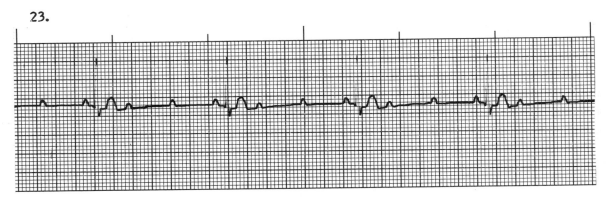

Interpretation of the above strip is:

    a.   Mobitz I
    b.   Mobitz II
    c.   Complete Heart Block
    d.   Sinus Bradycardia

24.   An appropriate intervention for the previous strip is:

        a.   Procainamide
        b.   Digoxin
        c.   Carotid massage
        d.   Pacemaker

25.

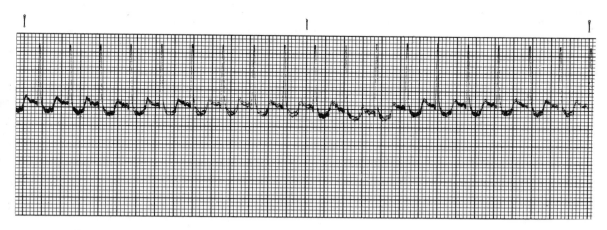

Interpretation of the above strip is:

        a.   Sinus Tachycardia
        b.   Ventricular Tachycardia
        c.   PAT
        d.   Junctional Tachycardia

26.   An appropriate intervention for the above strip is:

        a.   Digoxin
        b.   Atropine
        c.   Carotid massage
        d.   a and c

27.

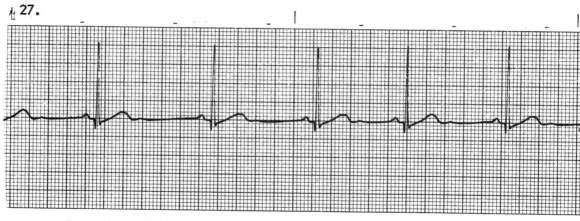

Interpretation of the above strip is:

    a.   Sinus Arrhythmia
    b.   Mobitz I
    c.   RSR with PAC
    d.   Bradycardia
    e.   a and d

28.   An appropriate intervention for the above strip is:

    a.   Atropine
    b.   Epinephrine
    c.   Carotid massage
    d.   Verapamil

29.

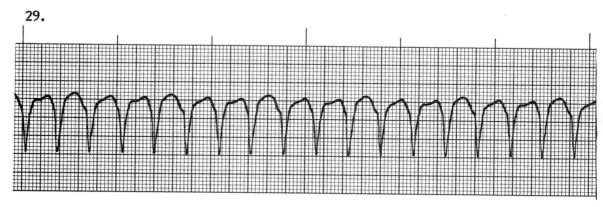

Interpretation of the above strip is:

    a.   Sinus Tachycardia
    b.   Junctional Tachycardia
    c.   Atrial Flutter 1:1
    d.   Ventricular Tachycardia

30. An appropriate intervention for the previous strip is:

   a. Verapamil
   b. Nifedipine
   c. Lidocaine
   d. Calcium Chloride

31.

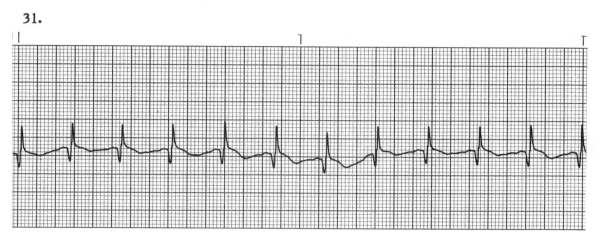

Interpretation of the above strip is:

   a. Junctional Bradycardia
   b. Junctional Escape Rhythm
   c. Accelerated Junctional Rhythm
   d. Junctional Tachycardia

32. An appropriate intervention for the above strip is:

   a. Epinephrine
   b. Isoproterenol
   c. Observe the patient
   d. Digoxin

33.

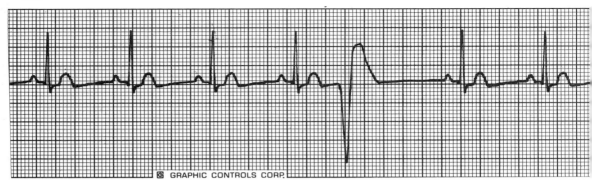

Interpretation of the above strip is:

      a.   RSR
      b.   PVC
      c.   First Degree A-V Heart Block
      d.   a and b
      e.   b and c

34.   An appropriate intervention for the above strip is:

      a.   Verapamil
      b.   Epinephrine
      c.   Isoproterenol
      d.   Observe the patient

35.

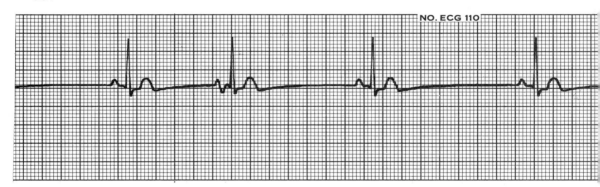

NO. ECG 110

Interpretation of the above strip is:

      a.   Sinus Bradycardia
      b.   PAC
      c.   PJC
      d.   a and b
      e.   a and c

36. An appropriate intervention for the previous strip is:

      a.   Calcium Chloride
      b.   Digoxin
      c.   Atropine
      d.   Bretylium

37.

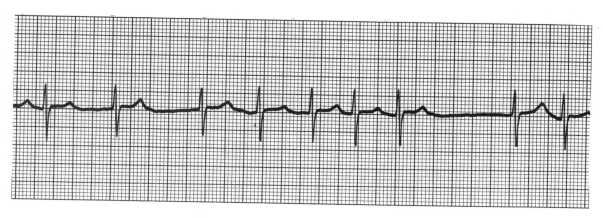

Interpretation of the above strip is:

      a.   Controlled Atrial Fibrillation
      b.   Uncontrolled Atrial Fibrillation
      c.   Controlled Atrial Flutter
      d.   Uncontrolled Atrial Flutter

38. An appropriate intervention for the above strip is:

      a.   Observe the patient
      b.   Atropine
      c.   Lidocaine
      d.   Carotid massage

39.

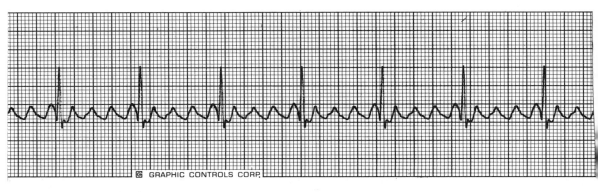

Interpretation of the above strip is:

    a.   Atrial Flutter
    b.   PAT
    c.   Sinus Tachycardia
    d.   Atrial Tachycardia

40.   An appropriate intervention for the above strip is:

    a.   Carotid massage
    b.   Observe the patient
    c.   Bretylium
    d.   Find and treat the cause

ANSWERS TO FINAL EXAMINATION

1.	c		21.	b
2.	c		22.	d
3.	b		23.	b
4.	d		24.	d
5.	e		25.	c
6.	d		26.	d
7.	a		27.	e
8.	a		28.	a
9.	d		29.	d
10.	c		30.	c
11.	d		31.	d
12.	a		32.	d
13.	e		33.	d
14.	a		34.	d
15.	a		35.	d
16.	c		36.	c
17.	a		37.	a
18.	d		38.	a
19.	b		39.	a
20.	a		40.	b